FROM ULTRASOUND TO ARMY

FROM ULTRASOUND TO ARMY

The Unconscious Trajectories of Masculinity in Israel

Hanni Mann-Shalvi

Primary Translator
Seree Zohar

Routledge
Taylor & Francis Group
LONDON AND NEW YORK

First published 2016 by Karnac Books Ltd.

Published 2019 by Routledge
2 Park Square, Milton Park, Abingdon, Oxon OX14 4RN
52 Vanderbilt Avenue, New York, NY 10017

First issued in hardback 2019

Routledge is an imprint of the Taylor & Francis Group, an informa business

British Library Cataloguing in Publication Data

A C.I.P. for this book is available from the British Library

ISBN 13: 978-0-367-10242-5 (hbk)
ISBN 13: 978-1-78220-081-9 (pbk)

Edited, designed, and produced by Communication Crafts

To my beloved
Assaf-Shmuel, Efrat-Bat Sheva, Ari Nahum, Alon,
Ella, Eden, Noam, Ethan-Moshe, Ophir, Ben and Gur,
with love, commitment, and gratitude

CONTENTS

III
Steps towards amelioration

ACKNOWLEDGEMENTS

First and foremost, I wish to express my admiration and thanks to the parents who opened their homes and hearts to me, sharing intimate thoughts and emotions. Their openness allowed me to begin to understand the secret processes accompanying parenting to sons in Israel, and the developmental stages in Israeli masculinity.

Completing this research and book was only made possible by the love, support, and emotional and professional involvement of several people, whom I wish to thank.

Two distinguished friends and colleagues, Salman Akhtar and David Scharff, opened the door to the professional international community and encouraged me to express my findings, thoughts, and understandings, both theoretical and clinical. I am immensely grateful to David for being a container in which my own development was enabled. I am filled with gratitude to Salman for his energetic and spontaneous manner, initiating the publication of this book.

Conducting my research in the framework of a doctoral dissertation at the Hebrew University, Jerusalem, was made possible by my mentor, Shmuel Ehrlich, whose support, guidance, and criticism led to clarification and consolidation of new theoretical understandings. My highest appreciation and gratitude to Eric King for his thorough editing of the English edition, caring for every detail and preserving the overall spirit.

Special thanks to Carol Gilligan of New York University, who gave generously of her time and experience to teach me the data analysis method she had recently developed, which allows raising unconscious levels to the surface. Many thanks also to Yoav Shiber, who helped me winnow the wheat from the chaff, shaping a study with an overwhelming amount of detail into lucid reading.

The research topic began with a very personal chord: from my deepest fears—of losing my sons in the army—which, up until this writing, I had been aware of only partially. Analysing the complex feelings expressed by other parents while removing defences from the text and being exposed to the difficult emotional dynamics that were only revealed while peering through the proverbial magnifying glass during analysis was a flooding exposure that became, at times, too difficult to bear. As a means of withstanding this emotional task, I shared tough as well as exciting moments with some people very close to me, whom I thank for their patience and tolerance.

Eitan Lewow helped me along my path by shining a torch into the darkest corners where elusive understandings hide. Eitan accompanies my life up close, warming the heart with his smile and creative approach. His very being and support has made so much possible.

My brother Haim Mann, who taught me how to handle the computer before delving into the sea of data. His unlimited accessibility and patience despite his full life as an attorney and businessman are deeply admired and respected. My dear nephews Amots and Ido Mann, and their friend Zak, my thanks for sharing your experiences as soldiers, enriching my comprehension and my writing.

My brother Udi, my brother-in-law Shlomo and sisters in-law Ella and Ruti, and Tali Alon, a friend as dear as a sister, who were always willing to listen, contain, and be there whenever needed.

Yoel, my children's father, who accompanied my life for thirty-five years and whose support and belief in me helped me stay dedicated to my task.

Last, but hardly least, my five children, who were my partners and my fan club throughout this long journey: Assaf, Ari, and Alon, who added their perspectives as combat soldiers; Efrat, who, though busy with her own doctorate, added her visual angle to the essence of the soldiers' image; and Ella, who has followed me into this field and was an enriching source of discourse.

This book is dedicated, with much pain, to the memory of my dear parents Moshe Yossef and Bruria Mann, and to the memory of my younger sister Sima Mann-ben-Torah, who passed away too young while this book was being written. Sima, artist and sensitive therapist, devoted and creative, woman, mother, sister, and aunt, was the epitome of a person able to integrate love of others with love of life and the world at large. I read parts of the book to her, an experience we both enjoyed. She will always be deeply missed.

And if family is our main topic here, let me end with a hope untypical of researchers: that for my grandchildren and great-grandchildren this study will be completely irrelevant.

ABOUT THE AUTHOR

Hanni Mann-Shalvi, who lives and works in Israel, is the tenth generation of her family in Jerusalem. She completed her doctorate at the Hebrew University of Jerusalem. She is a psychoanalyst registered with the Israel Association for Psychoanalysis, and her work is in couples and family psychoanalysis. She is Vice President of the International Association of Couple and Family Psychoanalysis.

She taught in the psychotherapy/psychoanalysis programme at the Hebrew University of Jerusalem and in the Israel Psychoanalysis Association and is an adjunct faculty member of its Child, Couples and Family programme. She founded and manages the international psychoanalytic couples and family training programme in Israel and has lectured at numerous international venues in Europe and in the United States.

As part of her doctoral dissertation, she has developed a research method called the Psychoanalytic Qualitative Research Method (PQRM), which uses psychoanalytic tools and understanding to explore unconscious psychic layers in society. Her method has been commended highly on the International Psychoanalytical Association's forum for psychoanalytic research.

Her teaching, research, and writing all employ psychoanalytic understandings to the complexity of unique characteristics in human identity, in existence in general, and in Israeli society in particular. Among diverse topics, she focuses on issues related to intergenerational trauma transmission in Israeli society. Her publications on this topic include "German and Israeli Jews: Hidden Emotional Dynamics" (in *The Future of Prejudice,* edited by Henri Parens et al.) and "Treating Intergenerational Trauma: The Bomb That Exploded Me Continues to Blow Up My Family" (in *Couple Psychoanalysis*, edited by David and Jill Scharff). The latter explores the unconscious dynamics occurring in families who have lost a family member through a terror attack.

FROM ULTRASOUND TO ARMY

Homo sum humani nihil a me alienum puto

Heauton Timorumenos, Act 1, Scene 1, by Terence, 163 BCE

In the spirit of "I am a human being, nothing human is alien to me", I set out on a journey that is reflected in the pages before you. It bubbled up like a fountain from the depths of my own psyche, around my many connections with my people, my country, my friends, and generations of family—my extended family and my nuclear family, my future family—and all that is different and unique in me. I set out to seek what we, parents of sons in Israel, undergo in these years that closed the twentieth and opened the twenty-first centuries.

Many of the emotional realities you will encounter as you read this book touch on deeply internal experiences and may not be the easiest of reading to digest.

Accepting in advance that we are all humans, with all that that entails, allows our curiosity to explore, with love, the encounters you will find when you join my journey.

Introduction

"If I cannot be myself in what I write, the whole is nothing but lies and humbug."

Ibsen, in a letter to Björnstjerne Björnson, 1865

The month of December. . . . Seven a.m., I am trembling inside, trying not to burst into tears. The pouring rain and grey skies echo what is happening within me. The whole family gathers around the door; my oldest son, Assaf, throws the large backpack that we packed the day before over his shoulders. "I shall be seeing him do this from tomorrow on for many mornings", I think, unbelieving, and we all leave for the induction centre.

This morning my firstborn son is being drafted into the army.

I stood with all the other tense-faced parents—the mothers red-eyed, looking at each other compassionately, with the camaraderie of mothers, the fathers' faces inscrutable. There was a spine-tingling silence, broken only by the voice of the announcer calling out name after name. I tried to dismiss invasive Holocaust associations from my mind. One by one, the boys—our sons—got on the bus. I felt as though part of my flesh was being ripped away, that I was doing something beyond my capacity, whereas in actuality I was not doing anything, just standing there like a statue. I could do nothing, only be strong, quieten all the fears, and say goodbye to my son with a smile and a blessing for the journey. The bus moved off into the distance; I hugged my children and my husband, and everyone went on their way. As raindrops mixed with my uncontrollable tears, I had a flash of insight: from the day he was born, the knowledge that one day I would have to let my son go to a place that endangered him "was there within me" and had resulted in a range of emotions the existence of which I could sense but not access, nor understand how they had influenced my mothering. The moment of my son's mobilization had accompanied me all the while I was raising him and his siblings.

From clinic to research: from individual to group

Over the years, this topic, which originated from my personal experience, echoed in therapy sessions with parents who repeatedly expressed the difficulty of setting boundaries for their children—particularly for their sons. The sentence, "I am really my son's friend", heard interchangeably as an expression of "good parenting", was accompanied by the giving of material things—expensive trainers, a car—that exceeded the parents' financial abilities and better judgement, silencing the authentic parental voice that guides and sets protective development-facilitating boundaries (Lewow, 2011). I met mothers whose childish pleading tone sounded as though they were trying to please their sons, fathers who did not dare voice their displeasure, and sons whose responses varied from childish to distancing, opaque behaviour.

When confronted with the dynamics of this relationship, the parents expressed feelings of being trapped, of unease, of guilt. They often attributed their difficulties to the fact of their sons' being pre-army, making it difficult for them to stop fulfilling their sons' desires because, "Who knows what will happen?" This attitude was accompanied by anxiety, resignation, and helplessness.

The reason for such a Catch-22 situation in parent–child relationships in Israel is the Compulsory Military Service Law for all eighteen-year-olds. Although the law applies to both men and women, only physically and mentally healthy men are drafted into combat units and therefore placed in potentially life-endangering situations.

Apparently, the parents' very knowledge that their sons are required to enlist and that their lives may be in danger is an emotional burden that affects and shapes parenting patterns. This awareness expands our understanding of the complexity of the processes that develop between parents and sons in the entire family unit: processes that can also result in similar characteristics in parent–son relationships countrywide and in patterns of masculinity and, accordingly, of femininity—that is, the unique patterns that characterize the army-serving society in Israel.

Although this topic has affected every family in Israel and intuitively seemed so relevant, I discovered that no research on it existed. I decided therefore to carry out an in-depth study of the topic, and the research findings and insights gained on the personal, familial, national, and international levels are presented in this book.

I hope that this book will let readers, irrespective of nationality, take an inside look at the inner workings of Israeli emotional reality, in a society founded on values of freedom and democracy on the one hand, but grappling with an ongoing existential threat on the other.

Preface to the research

The research question posited was whether the processes of parenting sons in the State of Israel are influenced by parents' knowledge of their sons' compulsory draft at the age of eighteen. This question shines a spotlight on a couple's approach and attitude towards parenting and the place that this information occupies in everything connected with their children and their own relationship—the influence of a future event, caused by the sociopolitical situation, on the delicate fabric of interpersonal relations and its effects in the child's emotional–psychological stages of development.

Via the research, I wanted to reach unconscious emotional processes hidden by what Freud termed "defence mechanisms"—mechanisms that, on the one hand, let us live by protecting us from being overwhelmed emotionally by the unbearable, but, on the other, often spoil our quality of life by hiding the way the past hurts and shapes in a limiting, disruptive manner our present and our future, subverting the achievement of our goals.

As an Israeli and a mother of sons, I was aware of the personal relevance of this topic. To ensure that the personal does not interfere with the research mindset, the researcher's personal involvement must be acknowledged. The associative thinking that, in part, motivated my research was that I wanted to "outwit" the disturbing defences—in the words of the Pharaoh—when he attempted to lessen the multiplication of the people of Israel by killing firstborns at birth. Actually, I wanted to do the opposite—to outwit the very influence of raising our children from birth in anxiety for their lives. Until I began to write, I had not realized I was still confronting the Pharaoh of thousands of years ago. A forgotten picture suddenly resurfaced from my childhood: playing Cowboys & Indians and making a blood covenant: cutting our fingers and mixing together the drops of blood. It was then I understood that perhaps the profound motive underlying my involvement in this work was the desire to unravel the tangled knots that tie generations to each other, with the commandment of memory, inscribed in "the spilled blood of your servant", the "blood libel" when we were accused of drinking the blood of the Christian child, "the blood of your holy servants", and the red blood of the Maccabees flower that grows in Israel and bears such a challenging, loaded name as a symbol for fallen soldiers and victims of terrorism. Perhaps this journey is meant to try to uncover the entangled bonds of hundreds of generations, to tens of generations, to the recent years, in the hope that we can rescue ourselves from their hold and become freer to try to build for our grandchildren a future that replaces the "blood, fire and pillars of smoke" with blue skies.

To achieve this complex mission, I relied upon knowledge accrued under the aegis of the psychoanalytic approach. Freud began the discovery of hidden and unconscious influences on our lives and the significance of basic drives as motives for our behaviour. His daughter Anna furthered his insight that various defence mechanisms come into play so that we are not overwhelmed by unbearably difficult emotional content.[1] Melanie Klein understood, in addition, the mother's important role in the child's emotional development. A number of theoreticians—the object relations school—believe that we are shaped by earlier relationships with our parents and driven by the need for relationships.

Despite the accessibility of this body of knowledge, I was surprised to discover that the worlds of research and of psychoanalysis had—perhaps for historical reasons—remained separate. I therefore decided to formulate a psychoanalytic research approach, based on qualitative research, that would facilitate focusing also on the unconscious level.[2] Through the research I was able to identify the formative influences of the knowledge of a son's future conscription on parenting and on the parents' relationships and also to understand the heavily laden ramifications for the maturation process of boys.

Part I of the book, "Developmental Backdrops", analyses the processes Israeli parents undergo upon discovering they will bear a son and the unconscious conflict that sabotages and shapes their parenting. This is a conflict the resolution of which is found in the couple arena, with the price of built-in tension in the couple's relationship.

Part II, "Vicissitudes of a Man's life", discusses the consequences of raising sons in conditions that encourage immaturity but foster hunger for masculinity. Other foci are the benefits and price paid for this reality by Israeli youth, and how they grapple with this challenging emotional and social demand.

Part III, "Steps Towards Amelioration", presents thoughts on how to apply these psychoanalytic insights to potential social interventions.

Although Israeli reality is depicted here, European and American society has faced similar situations during the periods of the World Wars, and these thoughts may therefore still resonate for some. The book also sheds light on the intergenerational communication of many in the Western world.

From Ultrasound to Army is being published simultaneously in Hebrew and in English—my hope is that its insights will open new channels of understanding and facilitate multilayered change through its contribution to dialogue, mutual awareness, and peace.

Notes

1. Defences are a group of psychic actions directed at reducing and minimizing any change that threatens the integration and stability of the individual's bio-psychological system (Laplanche & Pontalis, 1973, pp. 103–104).

2. The Psychoanalytic Qualitative Research Method (PQRM) is based on qualitative research accepted in the social sciences and approved by the Centre for Psychoanalytic Research of the British Psychoanalytical Society. The PQRM extends this qualitative-research study of the conscious layers derived, by studying the latent psychic layers, with the purpose of achieving deep familiarity with the people interviewed. The method enables recurring movement between emotional depths, revealed content, overview, and intelligence, while observing and auditing the data for documentation and review (Mann-Shalvi, 2007b).

PART I

DEVELOPMENTAL BACKDROPS

CHAPTER ONE

On learning the gender of the fetus

Preliminary investigation

Preliminary to my research on whether the thought of a son's anticipated/future conscription starts with awareness of the embryo's gender, I spent three days with gynaecologist and ultrasound expert Nili Yanai while she was examining pregnant women. Each time she told a couple they would be having a son, with permission I introduced myself as a researcher interested in their first thoughts on hearing of the embryo's gender. I did not mention my particular interest in parents and their sons, nor did I hint at any connection to conscription.

Ten couples were interviewed, and with each the men remained silent and the women talked about two worrisome events: circumcision, and enlistment into the army. One woman said, "It is wonderful that we have a son, but he will go into the army"; another said, "What immediately came to mind are circumcision and the draft." And a third said explicitly, "I wanted a daughter. I do not have the strength to cope with sons." To my question, "What don't you have the strength for?" she answered, "Primarily the draft into the army . . . it's frightening." There was something in the parents' eyes when they commented on the draft of he-who-was-still-an-embryo, as though from the few words, "He will be a soldier", I was meant to grasp all the hidden significance. As shown in this book, these code words encrypt all of Jewish and Israeli history.

My impression following the interviews was that the natural anxieties for the embryo's health were intensified and experienced as existential threats. Only after I had then undertaken and completed the research did I understand that these processes are also pervasive in almost every area of family life and in Israeli society in general and that they are fraught with intergenerational trauma. Consequently, public discourse on this topic is of utmost importance.

To be parents to sons in Israel

"To be parents to sons in Israel"—this sentence is replete with the complex emotional baggage that Israelis have carried since nursery school and elementary school: once a year, on Holocaust Day, the siren sounds and the country stands still, heads bowed in remembrance of the six million murdered Jews. Six days later the Memorial Day siren slices the air, and the Israeli world again stands still for a moment of silence in mourning for the fallen from wars and terror attacks ongoing since the state's establishment: in this way the bereavements of family and friends of the fallen are shared by everyone. The following night, on the eve of Independence Day, we stand again, trying to enjoy the colourful fireworks, whose explosive sounds again and again recall terror attacks or war.

An emotional world invades us and the hearts of our children: during the heartfelt nursery-school singing about Bar Kochba, whose character rides on the lion within us, "He was a hero/he called to freedom . . ."; in frightened wonder and admiration for the leader of the Jews in the revolt against the Roman Empire; in shock, hearing the stories of Masada, where 960 men, women, and children committed suicide so as not to give in to the Romans who blockaded them; listening, wide-eyed, to the stories and heroism of the one-armed Joseph Trumpeldor (his arm was amputated in 1920 during an Arab uprising, and he became a symbol of the willingness to sacrifice one's life for love of the Land of Israel). These and other stories join the Binding of Isaac, the Exodus from Egypt, the ten martyrs, and others, interwoven with values of courage and heroism, sacrifice of life for the sake of family, friends, society, faith, and longing for the Land of Israel, which over the years has often been replaced with loyalty to the state—all this in the face of a history of Jews being persecuted only for being Jewish, from the pogroms of the seventeenth century in Ukraine, to *Kristallnacht* in 1938 in Germany, and the Holocaust. Comprehension of all these mass deaths leads to *a pervasive anxiety that relentlessly seeps into the hidden layers of Israeli souls.*

Throughout our years at school, these texts and stories recur with different emphases. Our emotional platform is progressively created from within, and our parenting sprouts from these feelings. The same general components that intertwine with personal and family history create a unique and shared base.

Israeli history has been fraught with existential threats. To this historical base must be added a unique condition of Israeli life: at an age when many young people in the Western world leave the safety of home for university studies, Israeli youth begin army service: three years for men, two years for women.

The research

This story is woven together by parents whose sons were at significant crossroads in their lives in Israel at the end of the twentieth and beginning of the twenty-first century. The identity of the interviewees has been changed, but the spirit and message of their words has been preserved.

For the interviews, I selected twelve couples[1] in which both were either Israeli-born or immigrants to Israel before the age of ten years, and both had served in the Israeli army, and with sons or expecting a son and therefore able to anticipate the son's eventual separation upon conscription. They were interviewed either towards the end of the pregnancy, before the son started school, before the bar mitzvah celebration,[2] or shortly before the draft.

The interviews took place in the parents' home in the evening, in an intimate and quiet atmosphere that facilitated the free flow of feelings and associations. The parents commented that their hectic daily life did not allow for this sort of conversation.

To find out whether the son's future conscription would come up spontaneously in the interviews, I asked general questions regarding "thoughts and feelings accompanying child-rearing", without mentioning that I was focusing on sons or that military conscription and service were at the heart of the research. The conversations were open-ended, without guiding questions. Mostly, mothers spoke and fathers remained silent.

At the time of interviews (June 2000 to May 2003), Israel's security was in flux. The first interview took place just before the withdrawal of the Israel Defense Forces (IDF) from Lebanon following eighteen years of fighting. The general atmosphere in the country was one of relief and optimism. Other interviews were conducted in the post-withdrawal period, when there were numerous terror attacks, and there was a feeling of anxiety for one's life.

Unexpectedly, the emotional content of the interviews did not reflect that daily reality. In all interviews (except for one Israeli-born mother who had served in the army but had grown up in Europe), the sons' future conscription occupied significant space, starting with the thoughts accompanying the parents from pregnancy to birth, coupled with strong feelings of anxiety for their sons' lives during army service, internal and interpersonal conflicts, and behavioural strategies, some of which were not immediately discernible. For all parents, *the sons' future conscription aroused a flow of recurring emotional processes, usually in the same order.*

Careful listening reveals *a non-visible emotional reality, unique to Israeli parenting, that shapes patterns of parenting and relationships and also the identity of sons, and consequently of daughters, and thus profoundly affects the whole society.*

To my surprise, anxiety also came through as a formative factor in the couples' relationships, creating or escalating interpersonal conflicts. This process turned out to have ramifications for all areas of life, from the individual to the group.

On discovering the gender of the embryo

Ambivalence or "We are happy but . . ."

"*Mazal-tov* ["congratulations"]! You have a boy" is usually heard upon the baby boy's arrival in this world.[3] Given the unique place of a son in Jewish and Israeli culture, news of a son ought to be received joyously by the parents, but in all the interviews the parents expressed ambivalent feelings or thoughts.

As Ori, university lecturer and father of three sons, reported: "Purim 1983: the whole family was sitting down to the *seudah* [the festive Purim meal]. My brother called from the hospital to announce his son's birth. And what did he say? '*Mazal-tov*, a boy. August 2001!'"

Haim (well-known in cultural life in Israel), father of five sons, raised many eyebrows when he left Israel and, explained: "Every time they say, 'You have a baby boy,' I hear three knocks on the door . . . I cannot wait at the window for the next fifteen years . . ."—the three knocks being the army representative's knocks on the door to inform the family of a son's death, and waiting at the window for a son to return from the army—or the alternative.

These feelings are not only characteristic of the current generation; the earlier generation can be heard in the words of Lapid, father of two sons, who said in a tone of acceptance and identification: "Mother told us that when they came to Israel from Morocco, Father told her, 'The first two sons are my gift to the state.' They were different, our parents, from how we are."

Similar comments were made by parents of daughters: "When they told me I was having a girl, I was glad I would not have to deal with the issue of the army."

A doctoral student in the Psychology Department of Hebrew University called out during a lecture I gave, "Why didn't you start your research from the fertilization stage, when couples try to get pregnant and search for all sorts of methods to have a girl and not a boy because a boy will have to go into the army? I am at that stage of life . . ."

These feelings can be found in the media. Actress Limor Goldstein wrote in the *Ha'aretz* supplement (5 March 2004): "When I realized during the ultrasound that I was having a son, one of my first thoughts was how to lower his [medical] profile [so that he would not be in a combat unit]."

When I was writing this book, with one son in the army and two pre-army, I found the content of the parents' interviews difficult. To make things easier for myself, I searched for the "right" place to write. The Middle Eastern patio of the American Colony Hotel, located between East and West Jerusalem—a meeting place of politicians, diplomats, and journalists, Israelis, Palestinians, and foreigners—was one of my regular spots, as there I could experience what life will be like in Israel when there is peace in the Middle East, and thus I could deal with the overwhelming content.

Love in the shadow of the army: Sara and Sefi

I entered Sara and Sefi's home, and Sara welcomed me warmly.

Sara, young, pleasant, chubby, with smiling eyes, a soft voice and refreshing naiveté, was holding a baby, round like herself. She sat down on the sofa and her baby snuggled in, adapting his body to her curves. I felt as though I had been received into a warm, safe nest—a sensation that contrasted with the world shown in Sara's words. Her personal and family histories were intertwined with the army. As a young girl, she saw military conscription as an opportunity to escape from the Galilee village she was born into. She and Sefi met in the army; he was an officer in her naval coast radar unit. For Sara it was important to add that they had met under quite dramatic circumstances—not in the *Shekem*,[4] but when she identified a suicide boat that tried to enter Israeli territorial waters. They married a few months after their army service.

Sefi had grown up in a large family and wanted a large family, and Sara agreed happily: "I always loved children"; she willingly took on "the position of full-time mother". Sefi is the primary breadwinner.

I asked about their first thoughts after the children's births. They mentioned two of their three sons, completing each other's sentences. Sara began: "I remember that the thought of the army came up right away." I asked: "When? Where?" She looked at Sefi, who continued: "I think it was in the delivery room. When the oldest was born, we said, 'Wow what a bruiser' so as if . . .". Sara interrupted him and quietly explained: "Yes—in contrast with Gabi, who was born very small, and so we immediately said, 'The oldest will go to *sayeret matkal* [elite reconnaissance unit], and the second will be *shin gimmel* [guard at gate of an army base]'."

Like a bridge over troubled water: Naomi and Noah

Noah looked like an early-twentieth-century idealistic Marxist: a bookish man, lean, in khaki trousers and sandals. His whole being broadcast disdain for the emblems of the bourgeoisie. He told me that he had met his wife Naomi—tall, beautiful, curvy, vocal, and endlessly energetic—by chance.

The couple have a 6-year-old daughter, and they were expecting the birth of a son. Noah is employed by an international company and spends long hours at work. Naomi, who works in high tech and is a social activist in their communal settlement, entered the living room, laughing and apologizing for being late.

When I asked about their thoughts and feelings about raising children, she was silent. Noah answered in a quiet, helpless-sounding voice: "I thought when they told us we were having a boy . . . I don't know . . . that he is expected to go to a commando unit or something . . ."

Naomi ignored the distress in Noah's voice and declared aggressively that she would not let her son become a combat soldier. She clasped her hands over her stomach, protectively, and said that she was pregnant with a son. Something in her tone and evasive look made me uncomfortable. It seemed as though the joy and excitement of the impending birth had been replaced by fear of what was about to happen: "I am very tense about the birth. A son seems like a creature from another world. . . . In my opinion, boys leave mothers, while girls stay. . . . When I think about my son . . . I am afraid that he will be detached from the world, he will sit in front of the computer all day, and go 'Bang bang bang' . . . with those rifles, and when I ask him, 'How was nursery school?' I will obviously get a laconic, vague reply." She was sunk in thought for a moment, then continued: "In my heart, I knew that I would not get away with not having sons. . . . With time, I started getting used to the idea . . . but everything is still with . . . doubts." Naomi pulled herself together: "That is . . . *No*, I did *not* think that I would not continue the pregnancy because of this, *not* at all. As though . . . I will try to see him as something new . . . something I will learn to cope with."

Freud (1925) used the term "negation" for bringing up a topic via the negative. The word "no" cancels out the difficult emotional significance, protects the speaker, and gives a verbal outlet to thoughts that accompany difficult emotional content. One can therefore understand Naomi's intense emotional distress until thoughts even of stopping the pregnancy come up.

As though figuring this out on her own, Naomi said: "When I was very young, I already wondered what one does with all the energy, the aggression, Ninja-turtles, and swords of boys . . . Everything with boys is so tumultuous . . . I know . . . football . . . I don't know . . . my thoughts are not normal. . . ."

Only towards the end of the interview, after two hours of conversation, did Naomi return to the topic of boys drawn to football, and the not-normal thoughts suddenly had a different meaning: "In my opinion, boys have several things: football, cars, the army . . . this is what I said. He will have football and cars in his head, and then he will go into the army or something. . . . I don't know what happens, so. . . ."

She immediately pulled herself together, raised her voice, and announced to Noah that she planned to fight against the tendency to macho masculinity: "My son will not be macho, not with my upbringing. If Noah was someone who thought that he would take his son from the age of three to the stadium and push him into playing football . . . as though he clearly had a little buddy, that he takes and cultivates, I think I'd have to restrain that."

This picture of a mother who identifies masculine characteristics of her husband as potentially dangerous to her son's life, and therefore fights against her husband's male identity and her son's future male identity, including forbidding football games with the father, appeared in different variations in meetings with the parents, confronting a complex and problematic emotional reality.

We don't turn off the light at night: Galya and Gad

Galya grew up on a kibbutz[5] in the north in the 1960s. Her husband-to-be was a child on the same kibbutz. Her memories were of loneliness and emotional distress living in the communal children's houses, where all the kibbutz children slept together in rooms divided according to age. "I didn't want to sleep there. I would run away to my parents' home, and every time they would bring me back." She attested that in her childhood the rigid conformist framework dictated by the kibbutz experience was very difficult for her. She described nights of crying in the dark and alienation from the society of children. Gad, a year older than she, had similar experiences. When they met, it was obvious to them that they would leave the kibbutz and bring up their children with a totally different experience. "Children", she said, "have to be brought up by their parents and sleep at home and not with a caregiver in a children's house. We decided that we would not turn off the lights in the hallway."

I understood that very quickly their home had become a centre for their family, who loved to come and visit for a cup of coffee or a hot meal and pour out their hearts. One evening, when I arrived early, I smelt freshly baked cake. Galya's advanced pregnancy was apparent as she invited me to join Gad in the living room.

"A son this time, too", she said, without being asked.

My questions as to the thoughts and feeling accompanying the upbringing of their children were warmly welcomed. They were glad of the opportunity to speak about the most important topic in their lives: the upbringing of their children.

I was surprised by the openness with which they shared their disappointment upon discovering they were having a boy. The connection between their disappointment and their son's future conscription became clearer: "In the ultrasound, three doctors stood there with a new machine . . . and told us it was a girl. We were ecstatic . . . we wanted a daughter—we have boys, now we will have a girl. A month later we had another ultrasound and found out it was a boy. What a disappointment!"

Instead of happiness at the new experience, Galya found herself coping with the disappointment and the need to prepare for the birth of another son: "It took a while to get used to the idea. I had been sure I would fill the house with pink. I came home in tears. And then I went and bought two red shirts for boys—to change the colours in the closet—and that was it."

This is not an easy feeling prior to an impending birth. With effort, Galya repeated the words, "I'm ok" over and over, as though trying to convince herself and even force herself to feel this way.

Gad's matter-of-fact words were laced with anger and grievance and a feeling of "unfairness". "I . . . I did not need to separate from the pink things, I accepted it as it is. Although questions of chances and probabilities come up—Why four boys? Why does one of our friends have five girls, and another has three girls in a row?"

Galya and Gad did not connect their disappointment with their knowledge of the future draft. Based on their words, there was no reason to connect the dots. They detailed different wishes over their desire for a girl. During the rest of the interview, they spoke primarily about their anxieties for their children's well-being, but their underlying anxiety about their sons' future draft brings one to the likely assumption that the feelings are interconnected. In any case, if all Gad wanted were children of both sexes, why was he envious of his friends who only had daughters?

The perfect couple: Yasmin and Yitzhak

I met Yasmin and Yitzhak late one night in their attractive renovated house in one of the Sharon settlements in the centre of Israel. The easy flow between them was palpable. Married for twenty years, they work together in the family business and have four children, two girls and two boys. They clearly share a *Weltanschauung* based on the values of the importance of family life, work, and contribution to society. As common with families where values take centre stage, feelings were pushed into second place, and the focus was on overcoming weaknesses. From their words, I understood that their level of partnership was higher than that of most couples in their age bracket. They did many things together: working, going out, volunteering in various organizations. However, something in their relationship was discernibly awry: the conversation that evolved gave them the uncommon opportunity to share thoughts and feelings that did not usually have a place.

Very slowly, our conversation—which lasted until midnight—deepened, letting us touch on more complex, under-the-surface topics. Yasmin shared, at first hesitantly, memories of her fear when her son was born. Her body language broadcast a storm of feelings. She tried to continue speaking, and her movements transmitted what the words could not. She said, raising her voice emotionally: "I remember that when Eran was born, I was so afraid to love him. I was afraid that if

I love him, I won't love Becca—as though my heart wouldn't double but would divide in two. And that frightened me."

She was suddenly flooded with ambivalent, vague feelings. She caught her breath and continued in a somewhat childish voice:

> "I remember, I don't know how to explain it . . . It was most frightening. I really wanted another child. That is, not one of our children is an accident. But this I remember . . . In the beginning, the first two or three weeks, it was so difficult for me. I was so afraid to love him . . . It is not that I didn't hug him, kiss him, stroke him, so sweet, sweet . . . "

She was quiet for a second and continued in a tone that replicated her fear:

> "People ask: 'Nu, do you love him?' What can you say? No! I don't love him. It takes time until you . . ."

She lifted her voice and spoke slowly, exaggeratedly, to overcome the difficulty of saying these things:

> "When you . . . connect . . . to . . . this something that cries and yells and wants to eat and wakes you at night, and this . . ."

The intensity of her feelings overflowed in Yitzhak as well, who joined her as she struggled with words that refused to come.

> "I remembered here inside", she repeated, hand on her breast, "that it frightened me . . . that . . . if something happens to one of them, I will die."

The entrance of death with her memories of the beginning of her son's life, the ambivalence with which Yasmin's son was received into this world, with the anxiety for his life, resonate, although not directly, with the other couples. But this was only the beginning. As we will see, the anxiety for the children's life in general, and for the sons' life during army service in particular, did indeed take central stage in their relationship and parenting.

The couples we have listened to until now expressed ambivalence prior to the birth of a son, but they did not directly connect this with anxiety for loss of life during army service. One can infer the existence of this connection from the continuum of feelings—including the anxiety of loss and feelings of helplessness and guilt connected to the fact of the sons' future draft—that come up in all the interviews after the expression of ambivalence.

There were also couples who said clearly that they preferred daughters to sons, because they are not endangered in their army service. Let us meet two of them.

Girl, boy, girl, boy, girl, boy . . . Ruth and Rafael

The meeting with Ruth and Rafael was particularly heavy. It was as though they had waited for someone to give them a green light to begin to speak. I met them in their new home. Two of their sons were sleeping. Ruth was nursing her three-week-old son. I began:

> "The topic of this research are the thoughts and feelings that accompany child-rearing."

Rafael responded immediately: "The first thought is that they will go into the army. Especially since we have three sons . . ."

And then, as though stunned by the sharpness of his response, he added: "Very possibly, by the time we reach the army stage, none of this will have any meaning. But it is definitely the most frightening thing . . . when . . . you have . . . sons."

I asked about the birth of their new baby. For them, the entire issue had come up in her previous pregnancy, when they were first told the embryo's gender. The ultrasound technician had wrinkled her forehead, debating: "It's a girl . . . it looks to me like you have a girl." A deep sigh escaped them both. In the first pregnancy, they had also wanted a girl and had had a son. This time they were happy. "Our prayers were answered." When I asked why they preferred a daughter, Rafael answered: "Daughters manage better with the mistakes one makes with firstborns . . . they turn out better . . . Girls stay with their mother."

She described how through the last two months before the birth she imagined long conversations with her daughter: girl-time, someone who would be like her, a daughter totally hers. She then spoke about the birth: "I had such strong contractions, hours long, as though someone were ripping me apart inside. I was exhausted. But the birth itself was easy, smooth."

Ruth continued that when she opened her eyes, she heard, blurrily, the voice of the obstetrician announcing, in a happy post-birth voice, "*Mazal-tov!* You have a boy!!!" "We didn't believe it", Rafael said. We looked at each other in shock. "The midwife", Rafael smiled, "saw our disappointment and said, 'All the last births were girls . . . if you want, you can switch'."

Ruth looked into my eyes: "In the first moments I wasn't sure I would be able to love him, but when they put him on me and I felt his warmth on my body, I knew it would be ok."

They had called their firstborn son after a soldier who was killed in war. "I wouldn't do that today. I was too young. I didn't understand", Ruth said.

Their difficulty in this discussion was visible, their distress apparent in their fragmented speech, helping one another by completing thoughts and sentences. Anxiety for the life of a son, his future draft—from now on to be called "loss anxiety"—resounded in what their family and friends said:

> Ruth: "The name Roni was for our friend Roni, who fell in war . . . Our feelings swamped us almost immediately."
>
> Rafael: "The fear was that we would have a fighter. When we decided on the name, there were many opinions . . . around . . . because naming a child after someone . . ."
>
> Ruth: "No, it is not just after someone, but after a young person who . . . was killed in war . . ."
>
> Rafael: "The fear that fate should not 'catch' him as well, God forbid, when he is in the army . . ."
>
> Ruth: "There are all sorts of beliefs about this. For example, the critical age of the child . . . so when the young person is the age of the person who was killed, say twenty-one, that is a critical age for the person named after him."
>
> Rafael: "A sort of prophecy that shouldn't be fulfilled . . ."

The feeling of disappointment recurred in the second and third pregnancies when they discovered that Ruth was pregnant with boys. This time, Ruth said: "With Uriel, we were very disappointed. But we moved on right away. In the ultrasound."

Rafael gave additional details: "We kept saying, 'There can be mistakes in the ultrasound'." Then he laughed and said: "Then . . . then we took it bravely."

A division of roles *vis-à-vis* the anxiety accompanying raising sons developed:

> Ruth: "We discuss, I worry, and Rafael calms me down. That is our typical role-division in these discussions."

At this stage I was not yet aware that this was a couple dynamic that reflects the unconscious division of roles that develops between all couples in attempting to deal with the complex emotional load that accompanies the birth of a boy.

A pregnant woman naturally imagines how her baby will look; this is a universal and significant process for their future connection. During pregnancy, the mother's fantasies about the infant help her form ideas as to the baby's identity and personality and influence their developing relationship. Upon discovering the gender of the embryo, it is natural for the mother to experience, parallel with joy, the feeling of loss of an infant of the other gender, who will not be born. When a mother wanted a baby of the other gender, adjustment places heavy demands on her and can cause post-partum breakdown. In the post-birth stage, a great emotional and actual investment in the new baby is expected of the mother; this is different from her fantasies, and she does not have the time or emotional availability to work through the feelings of loss of the preferred child. The mothers who were interviewed related to the easier experience of mothering daughters compared to mothering sons. In Israeli reality, when parents cope with the loss anxiety associated with a baby boy, it seems that the coping with the loss of the unborn baby girl and accepting the baby that is born becomes more difficult and complex.

Mazal-tov! You have a soldier: Odelia and Oren

Odelia and Oren, who were both five years old when they moved to Israel with their respective parents, had grown up in solid homes with distinguished parents. Oren's father was a university philosophy professor, and Odelia's father was head of a surgery department and internationally known in his field. Their mothers were both involved in volunteer organizations. Their family life was tranquil, except for the tragedy when Odelia's cousin was killed in the Lebanon War. Oren has a distinguished position in a bank, and Odelia opened a successful sports studio. Their parents had jointly purchased an apartment for the couple, who had been married for two years.

I met Odelia and Oren in their home. Odelia's first birth became part of their memories of a fresh, new period. The interview allowed them special moments of sharing and open conversation with each other, something they had not had for quite a while.

When I asked about their first thoughts after the birth, Odelia answered in a contained, albeit angry tone. They had not known the baby's gender beforehand, wanting it to be a surprise. When the doctor announced that it was a boy, Odelia said:

> "My first thought was joy, regardless of gender . . . but then the midwife said with a big smile, '*Mazal-tov!* a new soldier is born.'"

This was the first time Odelia had shared these difficult feelings. Her words got stuck in her throat. In a voice filled with contained anger at the midwife, she said:

> "She got me into this . . . It was as if she said, 'Wake up Odelia, it is not going to be a honeymoon. You are bringing up a soldier here.' I was furious with her . . ."

Silent and sad, immersed in her thoughts, she continued:

> "From the moment the baby was born, the son was born . . . she had to tell me that . . . that you are raising . . . a son for the army. I remember that this made me angry and afraid. First fear, and then anger. And then with the second birth, already in the ultrasound they told us that it was a son, and I was upset."

Oren who had been quiet the whole time, expressed his feelings by quoting a friend's reaction:

> "I remember the third time I told someone who had just had a third son, and he said, 'Never mind. The next one will be a boy, and then you will have a girl . . .'."

If only the army weren't in the background, we'd be happy with sons: Ella and Eitan

The disarray in Ella and Eitan's house felt to me to reflect their lives: bicycles on their side, open backpacks with their contents on the table, along with dinner leftovers.

"Eitan will be right in", Ella said. She had just finished a meeting with her staff in the speech therapy clinic she ran, directing me to the kitchen table, clearing it quickly, preparing coffee for us. Upstairs, the TV sounds blended with those of their children: the oldest ten years, the second pre-school, the third three years old.

> "I allowed them to watch TV before they arranged their backpacks, so that we would have quiet", she said apologetically. Eitan came in, nodded hello, sat down quietly, and looked at me as though waiting for instructions.

Ella and Eitan radiated the desire to meet inner and outer reality without unnecessary defences and disguises. They listened curiously when I asked them to describe their thoughts and feelings accompanying child-rearing. Eitan began succinctly and openly: "From the first pregnancy, I wanted a girl."

Ella, who reported that she was usually very outspoken, found herself stuck and stuttering; hard put to find words for her feelings, she became confused with contradictory feelings:

> "In the second pregnancy we already had . . . that is to say, we were smiling, if . . . we would have been happy if they had told us that we had a daughter . . . don't misunderstand, we were happy when they told us in the ultrasound that we were having a son. That is to say, I was ready for another son, of course I wouldn't have been disappointed if it was a girl, but I was prepared and happy for another son . . . Of course I was happy . . . but the army is always in the background . . .

Not four sons! Not four soldiers: Dina and David

I met Dina and David, parents of four children—three sons and a daughter—shortly before their firstborn's draft. For the past ten years they had been living in a communal settlement, immersed in their satisfying professional tracks while concurrently trying to be involved parents. Dina remembered her firstborn's birth: "When my first son was born, I did not think about soldiers. Perhaps 'another soldier'. But it didn't sink in."

From a psychoanalytic point of view, some defence mechanisms for coping with the disturbing knowledge of the future draft can be identified. The first sentence, which raises the thought of the son as soldier that comes immediately with his birth, is said via negation. The use of negation (explained earlier in this chapter) lets Dina express her thought of the draft that awaits a son while simultaneously shielding her from anxiety about the new baby. The second sentence, "But it didn't sink in", also testifies to her need to protect herself from the terrible significance of the potential danger to her son's life. Via the process of dissociation, "she doesn't allow herself to know what she knows" (Gilligan, 2002). She then projects the feelings that are difficult for her to contain and express on to David: "David told me that when he heard that we had a son, he was a bit disappointed, because he thought I would feel badly, because he thought I wanted a daughter."

Dina's unequivocal happiness at the birth of her daughter stands in sharp relief to the birth of her son: "I was so happy that the second was a daughter . . . I prepared a blue list and a pink list; after the ultrasound I told David happily: 'Use the pink list'."

The connection between the youngest son's birth and the contents of loss showed up surprisingly: in their confusion regarding after which war they decided to have another child:

> Dina: "The fourth pregnancy was decided on after the Six Day War . . . no the Yom K . . ."
>
> David: "The Gulf War."
>
> Dina: "Yes, the Gulf War."

Their confusion is intriguing. In the Six Day War, they were in their early teens; at the start of the Yom Kippur War, in their army service; in the Gulf War, they were parents. One sees how the impressions and impact of the wars interact and intertwine from childhood to parenthood, creating complex emotionally laden baggage.

I asked: "What is the connection?" Dina continued in an uneven, quiet voice:

> "I felt that if we came out [alive] from this war, then I want another child. A frightening feeling . . . not knowing what is happening from now on. The beginning of . . . when they began with the missiles and all that . . . there was such a feeling of anxiety of . . . 'whether we will come out of this or not'. I said 'If we come out [i.e., if we are still alive], then I . . . want another child'."

And then she added, as though confiding:

> "If I had been promised another daughter, I would have had one right away. Not four sons, not four soldiers!!!"

When I asked when this thought came up, she answered:

> "About soldiers? When didn't it???"

Coping with their feelings was difficult for Dina and David. They "were helped" by projecting their wishes and anxieties on to one another. And so, when David "used" Dina to express his disappointment at the birth of a son, Dina "used " David, telling him: "If we had four daughters, you would be happy; we have friends with four daughters . . ."

> David: "I guess that would be ok."
>
> Dina: "What do you mean 'guess'? Of course it would be ok!"

Interestingly, Dina resembles Gad from the communal settlement in the Sharon who is married to kibbutz-reared Galya. For Dina (and for Gad) a preferable situation is one in which there are only *daughters*.

Knowledge of the future draft already hovers over and pervades the mother's complex emotional state of mind in pregnancy. At the end of the pregnancy and a few weeks after the birth, the mother is in a state of heightened sensitivity for her infant. She answers his needs totally, her boundaries merge with his. This role, according to Winnicott, is essential for creating the baby's emotional personality structure (Winnicott, 1956). It seems that the knowledge of the draft and the resulting anxiety for the loss of sons complicate the complex emotional picture, and thus *if the parents are ambivalent about the birth of a son, the loss anxiety makes it more extreme; if there is happiness first, the happiness becomes ambivalence.*

Shared emotions on a continuum

Mindful attention to the parents' words and body language and sensitivity to the unconscious messages reveal emotional positions that alongside the differences are on a surprising continuum, have a shared destiny, and reflect a range and richness of content and patterns of coping.

The parents' anxiety triggered a continuum of feelings that were expressed in thoughts and patterns of parenting. First, *ambivalence* when told that the embryo or infant was a boy.[6] Immediately afterwards came *anxiety for the lives of sons* during army service, accompanied with fear of bereavement and great difficulty. Expression of these feelings brought in its wake feelings of *helplessness* in facing an impossible-to-change reality and of *guilt* stemming from their need to protect their son's life. Their stories reveal the experience of bringing up life in the shadow of the fear of death.

There was unspoken cooperation as to "division of roles on the topic of children". In all the interviews in general, but more so when the couples discussed their sons' future mobilization, the mothers were responsible for the "children's file"—the primary spokespeople, the shofar of feelings, the leaders of the conversation who confirmed or encouraged the fathers to express themselves or contradict their spouses. The fathers cooperated in all the interviews; when the topic was their sons' future mobilization, the fathers were almost entirely silent. When they did speak, it was primarily in response to the mothers' comments, sometimes expanding them or adding a few words. Occasionally they opened their hearts and we had a peek into their closed world.

It seems that there are commonalities between the mothers and fathers, but with a great gap between them as well. After we listen to the mothers and fathers, we will offer an explanation as to why, unconsciously, the couples chose to divide the roles as they did, what the maternal and paternal functions fulfil in the family framework on the conscious and unconscious levels, and what the ramifications are for all the relevant circles.

Notes

1. See Appendix for details of couples who were not included in the research.

2. The coming-of-age ritual ceremony at age thirteen years in which they take on religious responsibility for themselves; it is also traditionally observed by secular Jews.

3. In Jewish–Israeli society, the birth of a son has unique emotional significance. A son says "*kaddish*" (a special prayer) after his parents' death and continues to carry the family name. In the biblical laws of inheritance, the firstborn son merits preferential treatment over his brothers, receiving a double portion, while the daughters receive nothing. After the birth of a firstborn son, there is a *pidyon haben* [redemption of the son] ceremony as a symbol and remembrance of the Exodus from Egypt. Circumcision is a symbol of the baby boy's joining the Jewish people. The bar mitzvah celebration—the ceremony at age thirteen in which boys take on religious responsibility for themselves—has religious significance, whereas until recent years the equivalent bat mitzvah celebration, for girls, did not. Men have more religious obligations than do women. Among the Sephardic community, the firstborn son is sometimes named after the father (who is alive) as a sign of honour and respect. Sons had especial status in the years of the establishment of the state.

4. Mobile canteen services.

5. A communal, usually agriculture-based, settlement unique to Israel.

6. A more detailed discussion on the connection between Israeli parents' ambivalence and ambivalence in the mother–infant relationship according to Klein (1946), Parker (1996), and Palgi-Hecker (2005) can be found in Mann-Shalvi (2005).

CHAPTER TWO

The mother's conflict

Through the window she looked, she peered—
Sisera's mother—through the lattice:
Why is his chariot so delayed?
Why do his chariot's wheels tarry?

Judges 5: 28

The Israeli maternal experience of sons

Mother's Voice has for over thirty years been the flagship programme of Galatz (abbreviation of Galei Tzahal), the IDF radio station for families and soldiers on duty. The Galatz mobile broadcaster visits bases across Israel, and the programme's presenter, Naomi Ravia, chats simultaneously with mothers and soldiers in the studio and conveys messages from families to the soldiers. The current study shows that the concept of "mother's voice" bears a significant and complex emotional message for Israeli families and society.

How is that maternal voice formulated? Knowledge of their sons' future recruitment seems generally to cause mothers a range of emotional and maternal patterns similar to those that consolidate a kind of shared yet uniquely Israeli maternal voice that expresses powerful anxiety over the lives of sons relative to their future military recruitment. These unique patterns are the topic of this chapter.

Maternal anxiety relative to future recruitment can flood the mother with complex emotions the intensity of which is difficult to contain.

Present in Israeli society's everyday life, they resurface particularly at times like memorial days.

It is important to keep in mind that the intensity of anxiety derives not just from the knowledge that recruitment awaits, but from multiple sources, some of which are, as we will see, unconscious.

The voice of anxiety

At the start of the interview, I asked parents a general question on "the thoughts and feelings accompanying you as you raise your children", adding nothing further. The mothers themselves spoke up, like Dina, who immediately answered:

> "I'd like to say that happiness is the strongest, that I couldn't imagine my life without them, that they teach me and add so much. But I actually start with concern, because it's the basis of what will accompany me into the future, my son will soon be recruited into the army . . . my son . . . he's being recruited . . .!"

Hedy was no less direct. Tenth-generation residents of Jerusalem, Hedy and Hillel presented themselves as "typical Jerusalemites". Hedy teased Hillel that his clothes were always the same few items, that he'd never switch from his childhood barber, doesn't express emotion, isn't a romantic. He'd toss back that she's much like him about clothes and also has a direct approach. Hedy, a former basketball team member, has kept her athletic appearance. She spent her army service in a kibbutz and after her compulsory duty stayed on for five more years. For both, family and their sense of belonging to, and being responsible towards, the country are second nature and the foundation on which they established their own family, now numbering two sons aged six and seven, and a third about to be born.

The interview took place just days before the IDF evacuated from Lebanon in May 2000, a move that aroused stormy public discourse and created an atmosphere that swung between euphoria and deep worry. Hillel said that he didn't "think about the anticipated danger to his little boys of being in the army in the future", but Hedy protested strongly:

> "Well, you've adopted a political stance that sides with the IDF leaving Lebanon, even though it negates your real political views, only for the sake of not having your kids in Lebanon . . . you told me so, clearly. Well, of course . . . would it be better for them to get killed?"

Sign language

Most of the mothers were unable to express their fears as clearly as Hedy, but they found a range of alternatives, a kind of socially accepted sign language. Most spoke hesitantly, starting and stopping, overcoming the emotions flooding them. Some expressed themselves through allusion, code words, body language, silence, or unfinished sentences, letting the listener complete their sentences.

Ruth and Rafael look like siblings. Tall, slim, with blue eyes and light-coloured hair, they convey sadness and gentleness to me. Both opened up about the fear of losing their sons in the army. Ruth, breast-feeding her newborn during the interview, said that "the questions are really being raised", but when she tried to share what they were, she was unable to complete sentences: "Yes, I . . . Rafael, what will be? And if . . . God forbid . . . What would we do . . .? How would we cope . . .? We're asking all those questions."

Another way mothers found of alluding to their feelings was to say that they're *scared*, adding little or nothing further. Dina, whose son would soon be recruited, said, "I think about how, at eighteen, they're recruited . . . it's scary." Yasmin, mother to three sons and two daughters, also noted that "If he goes to Golani[1] . . . I know it will scare me, that I won't sleep at night because of it, that I'll be worried."

Becca's parents had immigrated to Israel from Morocco. They wanted to give their seven children the best they could, despite their meagre income. Becca decided that she would have only a small family but, like her parents, would try to give them the best of everything. Boaz, her husband, came from a similar background. When they met after their military service, it was as though they had found their soulmates. At the start of the interview, Becca remarked how, from the moment her sons were born, her heart filled with concern for their future lives in the army. Using the word *"fears"*, Becca added, "it's clear what fears I mean":

> "There are fears. For three years there'll be fears. The fear that it's a month until my son's recruited, my fear . . . that nothing can be done about it. Recruitment was supposed to have been in November, so we said ok, he's got another half year with us, but then they moved it forward to July . . . and the butterflies in my stomach flap harder . . ."

Yasmin offered the commonly used term in Israeli society of *"if something happens"*:

> "You want to give your kids everything you can before . . . anything happens to them . . . because if something happens . . . truthfully, it's scary. Recruitment itself isn't scary, the scary part is if there's a war, and if things carry on the way they are now, and if it doesn't end, and it's scary that something could happen to my children . . ."

"Combat" raises images, myths, and traits that are among predominant components in the makeup of the Israeli male identity—courage, power, self-confidence, daring, resourcefulness, values, willingness to sacrifice, poise, solidity, and pride. But it naturally also encompasses anxiety regarding the young man's life.

> "I think these fears will last the whole three years . . . he wanted either a combat unit, undercover, or Duvdevan[2] . . . they told us it's a combat recruitment—Golani, Givati, or tanks, that's the fear. Peace hasn't come yet. There's fear. You hear so many incidents, every day a soldier's injured, those are the fears . . ."

The phrase "*lose your son*" replaces a more explicit statement, as in Galya's words: "I don't want them to be combatants. I don't want to lose them."

As a collective associative phrase, "*the last trip*" is the way bereaved families often describe their sons' last civilian activities before they fell in combat. Dina said:

> "We took a trip to Belgium in the summer. I made this trip bec . . . because . . . I don't want to say 'last trip' but I had this thought that should anything happen, then the trip would . . . and . . . and . . . I wanted us all to have this really good experience before . . . before the army . . . so of course these . . . the thoughts went through my anxious mind that it could be the la . . . the last trip . . . we take together. But . . ."

Her pain could be heard as she continued:

> "But to them I explained that it was the last trip be . . . before going into the army, afterwards they'll probably travel with their friends . . . it's . . . it's something that really . . . I did it very consciously."

Her husband David nodded. A tear fell from her eye, and they both remained silent.

After some two hours of conversation, with a growing sense of intimacy among us, Dina felt more comfortable with sharing thoughts that, until that point, had remained closeted in her mind:

"I don't know if . . . I mentioned this. A thousand times . . . I imagine the moment . . . how they inform . . . so many times . . . I never even raised it here, because it's so difficult . . . it's not that I didn't want to talk about it but . . . it's hard to say it out loud to yourself so exactly."

Dina gazed at me with a look that I interpreted as a mingling of pain over the subject matter with relief for having shared her secret.

The labyrinth of unresolvable maternal conflict

These maternal statements, accompanied by intense emotions, exemplify expressions that recurred throughout the interviews. Even today, I meet mothers who express themselves in very similar ways. Without any connection to the state of security in Israel, or to the age of their sons, mothers detail their sense of real despair and almost life-paralysing anxiety over the lives of sons who will be recruited.

The reasons behind the depth of the anxiety expressed by mothers are not anchored in reality: injuries sustained while on military duty are not the main source of injuries among young Israeli men, as is detailed in chapter five. In fact, the numbers of traffic accident injuries and deaths are far higher than those of losses due to war. It seems, then, that fear of combat service is not the real source of anxiety over losing their sons: analysis of the interviews revealed other reasons for maternal stress.

It is not military service per se that holds mothers in an emotional trap that impairs their ability to function, but, rather, the knowledge that accompanies the act of parenting boys who could be recruited into activities that may endanger their lives.

The role of mother encompasses a dual task: that of raising sons confidently towards healthy lives while allowing them to develop their individual masculine identity separate from the mother. For her son to grow into an independent man with a defined, developed sense of self, the mother needs to accompany his gradual grasp of independence and tolerate the emotional space that will allow separation from a close, intimate relationship with her (Bowlby, 1988, p. 12; Chodorow, 1978). The fact that by law every physically and mentally healthy male must, on reaching the age of eighteen, enlist for combat service creates a situation where these natural maternal tasks contradict each other: a mother who successfully raises her son to independence and manhood will see him given the highest conscription evaluation—"97 profile"—none other than a combat rating. He will most probably be recruited into a position where his life could be endangered. For a mother to prevent this destiny and protect her son, she needs to keep him beside her in a state of dependence, and to negate the maternal role of allowing her son to become independent—a masculine Israeli man.

In successfully fulfilling one maternal task, the mother fails in the other. Unaware of this source of her anxiety, she relates it to the fact that she fears for her son's life. Mothers who found themselves needing to choose between these two tasks opted to protect their sons by keeping them close, sometimes at the cost of sabotaging the masculine individuation developmental process.

Before exploring the parallel process undergone by fathers and manifestation of these conflicts in the couple's relationship, let us take a closer look at maternal feelings—especially the ways in which they shape the norms of motherhood over the course of their sons' lives.

Helplessness and lack of control

Helplessness and lack of control were the intense sensations expressed by mothers because of their inability to protect their sons and save them from the dangers inherent in military conscription. Surprisingly, these sensations recurred without any relevance to sons' ages—evidence that the sources of these emotions are not anchored in the concrete reality of recruitment. Becca, whose son would soon be drafted, defined the feeling well: "The feeling is that it's an edict."

During pregnancy, the foreknowledge of raising a son already gives rise to the sense of a clock ticking, marking the encroaching threat to the son's life. The army is experienced as the most extreme situation of absence of control, and so the natural development of gradual release of the adolescent son is perceived by the mothers as a process with which they are not willing to cooperate.

Naomi, for example—who was nearing the end of pregnancy and carrying a son—completely ignored the fact that when her son reached a certain age she would no longer be able to dictate to him how to conduct his life; she asserted in a very formidable tone: "I won't send him to the reconnaissance unit!" Noah, noting her comment, chuckled as he said, with some sadness: "At eighteen . . . he won't be asking you."

Perhaps her statement can be put down to lack of experience. But Galya, mother of grown children, to whom it is clear that these developmental processes will come about even if they are against her wishes—that for the sons at age thirteen, as part of the normative process of growth, the peer group becomes more significant than parents (Esman, 1985)—also expressed herself similarly:

> "It looks so complex! These youths . . . from thirteen you can't solve things by force, not even when you scream . . . my son's stronger physically and with his words . . . how he answers me. They no longer snuggle up to you, they've got their own crowd . . . I'm losing control, and all you've got is what you gave them up to then . . ."

Not only does Galya have trouble being glad that her sons are developing, but that same development is, for her, tied to her inability to control the lurking dangers.

> "I don't trust the army . . . To me it isn't heroic to participate in . . . in terrible battles. I wouldn't want my kids to get to that, even though I don't think I'll have control over it, and I'll just have to let them choose what they want because they'll be grown up."

The sense of guilt

In all the interviews, the mothers expressed guilt feelings over not being able to fulfil their duty of both raising sons securely and allowing consolidation of their separate male identities.

The psychoanalytic approach, especially Melanie Klein's, views guilt feelings as part of psychic development. These emotions arise when the infant begins to realize that the world, including the mother, is not separated into good or bad but that within every person—and, later, within every situation—there is a connection between the two. Once infants can integrate these two experiences, they begin to understand that while they are not perfect, they are not only evil. Later this understanding will encompass their loving parents and, as time goes by, other situations in their lives.

Such perception is vital for understanding the complexity of life, developing the ability to deal with loss of a loved one, coping with situations where loved ones hurt us in some way, and accepting the destructive parts within ourselves. These two emotional stances—splitting the good from the bad and integrating the two—continue to accompany us throughout our lives. Occasionally, when we are flooded with forceful emotions, we find it hard to contain both the "good" and the "bad" within us and may find ourselves again looking at the world in terms of black or white. Transitioning from splitting of good from bad to emotional integration—a complex reality with both advantages and disadvantages and accompanied by guilt feelings, pain, sorrow, and the wish to correct and compensate (Klein, 1937a)—is a universal developmental process. Apparently the Israeli reality, in which a mother who raises her son to have high emotional and physical capabilities leads him into danger when he is conscripted, results in stronger maternal guilt feelings.

Emotions that are difficult to contain and express in a moderate way become a source of disruption in personal relationships. Guilt feelings fit that bill perfectly. Here are comments made by Sara, Dina, and Odelia, the only mothers who described their guilt feelings openly. As Sara said: "It's important to me to be involved in my sons' lives, so that I won't later say . . . that I sat by with folded arms and did nothing, so that I'll know I did what I could to protect him and keep him safe."

Dina said that "It's not natural to go to a movie or coffee shop, and they're . . . in the army. For three years I won't travel overseas, because what if something happens just when I'm not there? But these are really guilt feelings—how can I truly enjoy myself at a time like this? It's tough."

Odelia, who had immigrated to Israel when very young and who has young children, shed light on yet another angle: "Because I wasn't born here, another option is open to me that, if I chose it, would see my sons not being conscripted. I constantly feel guilty about being connected to Israel . . ."

Most of the mothers were unable to bear the guilt feelings and projected them onto their husbands. The only mother who described this openly was Leah. She blamed Lapid: because of his educational approach, the values he inculcated into his sons, and his refusal to leave Israel when their son received his first call-up papers, he is perceived by her as directly responsible for their son being recruited to a combat unit. She added: "I let him decide, and I played the simpleton. That releases me from responsibility. Later . . . I can direct my complaints to him. He knows that."

This issue—as we will see—runs like a silken thread through the fathers' emotions and the couples' relationships.

There's no love like a mother's love

The topic of a mother's love— the conscious and unconscious erotic sensations between mother and child—is taboo outside the psychoanalytic clinic. The term "erotic" is not actually apt here, since it relates chiefly to sexual sensations, whereas the raw sensations aroused between mothers and their children are termed "libidinal" and are linked to the life urges and sensuality. The latter also encompass sexuality.

Psychoanalysis acknowledges the existence of libidinal sensations arising in the mother towards her infant, particularly following birth and during breastfeeding, but also later, as life progresses. They are considered an important part of psychic development. A mother is, first and foremost, a woman. The processes of coition, pregnancy, birth, and breastfeeding involve erogenous zones and occur simultaneously with significant hormonal changes.[3]

Interestingly, this aspect, to which many give no thought in the context of parents and children in general, and mothers and sons in particular, is referenced in ancient Judaic sources by way of a prohibition: "None of you shall approach to any that is near of kin to him, to uncover their nakedness" (Leviticus 18, p. 6). Rambam[4] provides the explanation that it is prohibited to enjoy forbidden incestuous contact at the sexual level, as well as without actual sexual relations:

> This warning we have cautioned: against enjoyment of any of the incestuous relationships, even without intercourse, such as hugging and kissing and other related actions that a person enjoys.[5]

Again, we can learn of the existence of this sensation through its prohibition.

Relating to the father's sexuality during the breastfeeding stage, Palgi-Hecker (2005) notes that the breastfeeding mother faces, perhaps for the first time in her life, a difficult conflict, which pitches her against the incest taboo. The sensations of giving, providing, concern, and more—all these being maternal feelings—mingle with the erotic pleasure produced by breastfeeding.

Young (1990) reported that many mothers resolve this dilemma by denying, or alienating themselves from, such sexual pleasure or, conversely, by foregoing breastfeeding because it arouses their disgust. The mother is then required to find a new order within herself, or a new continuum between her own familiar eroticism and the new motherhood-derived eroticism. The sources of her erotic sensations are her psyche and body and are based on touch. How, then, can the mother distinguish between the different sensations (Palgi-Hecker, 2005)?

Whether conscious or unconscious, this is not a simple psychological issue to cope with, and for Israeli mothers the unique conditions surrounding motherhood increase the complexity: on the one hand, they make it possible to acknowledge the psychological complexity;

on the other, they further complicate psychological coping for Israeli mothers of sons.

I found that fear of a son losing his life surfaced in very early stages of motherhood, causing the image of the newborn to be viewed as a combat-soldier-in-the-making: the prototypical Israeli male, a sexual male figure able to arouse imaginary sensations of attraction and desire. These feelings may confuse the mother and be perceived by her as prohibited.

During adolescence, when the son becomes a man, the processes of separation typical of this stage make it easier for the mother to cope. In contrast, during the early stages, when the relationship with her son is one of fusion, even an imaginary encounter with her son as the ideal male is far too early, confusing, and flooding: not suited to her developmental stage as a mother and to the infant's as her son, such sensations will naturally be repressed into her unconscious.

In a well-known Israeli song, *My Haimkeh*, maternal love out of sync with reality is sketched out with humour, starting with a mother's surprise at the masculinity of approaching soldiers, all wearing military berets, with their badges facing front. The song describes the mother trying to neutralize the erotic aspect in her amazement at her son's physique by relating childishly and forgivingly to the difficulty of his integration into the masculine marching rhythm:

> Only my Haimkeh—his badge is turned to the back!

When the mother has calmed herself down with the thought that her son isn't like his mates, a tough muscular guy, she calls him "sweet", using a word reserved for children, not for men. This sets her free from the difficulty of separating from him and her wish that her son will continue expressing his love publicly only for her:

> Only my Haimkeh calls out, "Hey, Imma,[6] it's me!"

And she repeats the message that, indeed, "Only Haimkeh loves his mother always." Dina, whose son is about to be recruited, echoes this, her stammering evidence of her hidden discomfort: "When I think of soldiers, in addition to the values, there's that element of manliness . . . ever since I was a teen, soldiers always seemed to me . . . even now I connect to that feeling . . . that arouses pride. I'd like him to succeed . . . but on the one hand we're very scared, and on the other, you want . . ."

Dina and Yasmin were shaken by anxiety and guilt over the longing to see their sons as men, yet turn them into boys. Dina said: "I *am* proud of the kids who are doing things, reaching positions of command. Yes, it's still the image of the . . . of the goodly Israeli . . . he'll be going soon . . . to protect me there, so can I tell him when to go to sleep?"

Yasmin wanted her son to be a "Shekemist",[7] a non-combatant soldier who sells sweets to the combatants, and added: "It'd be nicer for me . . . no, actually, I'd die of shame . . . it's a tough conflict because you don't want anything to happen to your kids. Not even when protecting the country you love so much . . . and it's not important to me what others think about me . . . nonetheless I'd die, that it's my son . . . and he's not a fighter . . ."

Leah's love sounds like true couple love under the guise of loving an infant: "He's so attached to me, and he only wants me, and he won't give that up. And I'm telling you, Sunday at the recruitment centre, the first thing, he'll phone me."

Then she mimicked him, in an indulgent voice: "Imma, make this for me, and this, and come here to me, and write for me, and I love you . . ."

Keeping sons attached serves both the maternal wish to protect them and the forbidden attraction. This, as we will see later, is an emotional dynamic with far-reaching consequences on couplehood, femininity, and masculinity.

When a son starts school

A child starting school is a significant developmental stage in the life of the whole family: all are challenged and involved in redefining positions and roles (Gould, 1975; Levinston, 1986; Sheely, 1976; Silverman, 1982).

The mothers interviewed experienced their sons' start at school as another stage in distancing from them and approaching the military danger that would threaten their lives: a transitioning from the protected environment suited to their sons' needs and under their control to a system of rules and boundaries where their control is limited. They transferred to the schools the feelings in their hearts towards military service, relating to both in the same breath. As Sara said:

> "Up until they're five years old, we're used to accompanying them everywhere . . . then suddenly you need to send them to school, and mentally you need to let them go . . . it was really hard for me to release them into school, to send them. Every morning I'd say 'May light and love go with you', and I say to friends who've got

> sons in the army, 'If you're worried, send them light and love, and then you'll be calmer, and they will too.' . . . I have no other choice. On the one hand, I think that maybe we don't have to send them to school . . . But now I see it's not so terrible, maybe I can send them to the army and then see it's not so terrible."

Ella, Ruth, and Odelia also referred to school and the army in the same breath. Hostile towards school in advance, they saw it as an anonymous system that doesn't relate to the individual, is not attentive to individual needs or difficulties, and endangers an individual's health—as a place of violence and of unreliable teachers. Not a word of praise was heard, only anger and frustration. Here is what Ella said angrily as her hands carved out large movements:

> "This child is not the country's *and not the army's,* he's mine and my husband's and his own. *And I don't rely on this army at all!* If I could choose not to comply with the law so that he wouldn't get hurt, I would . . . *and I've got the same lack of confidence towards the school.* But *with the school I have some level of control."*

She enumerated similarities with the army, as her voice grew increasingly louder:

> *"In the army,* kids are handling things: a child about a year older than mine is his commander and takes fateful decisions, and I don't feel good about that . . . I . . . I'd really like to rely on that system. But the reality, the newspapers, and my own service prove otherwise . . . *the army* can take from me, and I don't . . . and again, it *links with the school,* a framework with rules where sadly people making decisions are hardly the generation's great luminaries, but politicians who don't understand what education is. The teachers behind their desks are mostly not smart women . . . and they can destroy a lot of what's important to me . . . values, decency, courtesy . . . the only reason I'm willing to send my son to school is that at school at least he won't get hurt physically . . ."

Then anxiety and anger flooded her:

> "Bloody hell, *who are you, army, who do you think you are?* He's my child! I understand that you've borrowed him, but you can't take from me all the connection I have, I can't just put him aside for three years, you've got no right to do that. *The same thing with the school.* Things that happen at school . . . and Nadav's in third grade and already knows how to say that he hates school . . ."

Ruth spoke in a similar way, the anxiety over whether her son would hold up leading her to a dilemma:

> ". . . how involved to be, or not be . . . school is really hard for us . . . and of course I'm also thinking about the army."

When taking these feelings into account, it is easy to understand how the mothers feel that their sons are fledglings and too tender. As Ella said:

> "He's just a *fledgling* . . . my anxiety is over him not cooperating because he doesn't like to do things he doesn't enjoy . . . I'm afraid that he won't manage, because the system doesn't support lack of attention."

Or as Odelia said, echoed by Ruth, who used exactly the same words, "He's a really, really *sensitive* child who loves to play all day."

Anger and lack of trust in the education system—feelings that may have some basis in reality—make the mother hostile towards the system. Natural developmental difficulties in the child are experienced by the mother as confirmation of her feelings. Clearly, these messages are passed on in overt and covert ways to the sons (detailed further on). Awareness of this dynamic sheds a different light on complaints of many teachers concerning parental over-involvement that sabotages the school's regular proceedings.

The transition from nursery school to school was identified as a worsening of circumstances and the desire to protect their sons, distance them from pain, pamper them, keep them close at hand. This wish arouses conflict, since mothers know that if they behave this way, their sons will not be ready to cope with the tough conditions they will need to face when serving in the army—a wish, they understand, that endangers their sons even more. Odelia describes it as follows:

> "Ever since they're little I've struggled with *how much I need to prepare them for army service.* They were happy in their lovely nursery schools, with a few other children, and I felt good because they were protected . . . from bad people . . . they weren't shouted at, their internal worlds were reinforced and enveloped."

Odelia's use of "bad people" demonstrates how a specific threat anchored in future recruitment turns into an amorphous threat accompanying life's progress and hence plays a central role in choosing the school to which the sons are sent. Her fear that her son, who has attention deficit disorder (ADD), may not find his place in the army was solved by deciding to send him to an arts-based school so that ". . . they can educate him not to go to the army . . . and then it'll be his decision".

The link between entering school and future recruitment demonstrates how deeply the Israeli mother carries the image of her son as a combat soldier in her psyche, even if unconsciously. Since in Israel the combat soldier represents the Israeli man (Sasson-Levy, 2006), the mother finds herself in an emotional duality, shifting between her experience of him as the ideal, omnipotent combat male and her feelings towards him as the helpless, vulnerable fledgling—polar images that do not allow her to relate appropriately to her son's developmental stages. We can thus understand how she does not acknowledge the child's otherness but, instead, perceives him as part of herself, of her body.

There is a connection with the libidinal claim: whether the son is a vulnerable infant or the tough fantasy partner, there is no realistic differentiating perception of him. The symbiotic fantasy is shared by the longing to return her son to the womb, and thereby void the world outside them, and the sexual-romantic ultimate fantasy of fusion and assimilation. The sense of irrational guilt in the mothers' statements surfaces over agreeing that their children would go to school: the experience they express is as though something has been torn from their bodies, indicating that the mother does not acknowledge the child's alterity and perceives him as part of her, part of her own body. The difficulty of emerging from this symbiotic relationship is noticeable.

As bar mitzvah approaches

Adolescence, a period of transition and change accompanied by emotional tempests, affects both teenagers and family. The adolescent copes with issues of identity building, consolidating the experience of self, shaping the social self, psycho-sexual development, and developing the ability to separate and individuate (Blos, 1962; Erikson, 1950; Freud, 1915a; Winnicott, 1971). The relationship between mother and son undergoes similar changes. It is therefore of concern to encounter mothers of sons approaching adolescence who describe their sons in the same words as mothers of much younger sons.

Yasmin and Yitzhak, successful business owners who convey a sense of capability and control, are parents of a son approaching bar mitzvah, a daughter of fifteen, a son in secondary school, another in primary school, and a toddler daughter.

Yasmin is in her early forties, energetic and vital. She articulates quickly and describes herself as involved in her children's lives, careful about their education, and very protective, especially of her sons, with whom she conducts an "endless" battle aimed at ensuring they invest in their studies. Every refusal on their part makes her feel pressured: "With Roi, I have a daily battle over his music: 'Roi, practice playing,' 'Not now, soon, later . . . I played two days ago . . .'"

At the same time, she worries about her attitude and whether she is harming her sons: "I often ask myself if I'm not 'pillaging' something from my children by being so pedantic with them . . . it always bothers me, whether I'm doing the right thing, because the way we raise them influences their futures."

Yasmin's verbal ability is impressive, her voice is clear, her words well enunciated, her laughter fills the room. Her busyness at many levels leaves the impression that she has successfully overcome her doubts and created a maternal pattern of confident potency. Listening only to the overt content in her remarks gives no hint whether they represent the true situation.

Carol Gilligan (2002) developed a technique—the "I-Poem"—that allows listening to the covert layers in interviews by extracting the word "I", and the verb following it, from the whole sentence and using them to structure a sequence of statements that look like a "poem of me". This brings to the surface the otherwise hidden emotional reality. Listening this way to Yasmin's comments makes the scope of her anxiety accessible:

I mess up (my children)
I don't let them
I don't let them
I mess them up completely
I don't let them
They'll turn out terrible monsters
I know
I see
I argue
I don't know if I'm doing the right thing

With the original negation removed, the symmetrical structure—opening with the harsh sentence "I mess up my children" and ending with "I don't know if I'm doing the right thing", as well as the frightening thought of "they'll turn out monsters"—speaks volumes.

And I don't know
If I'm doing right or not
I do
I give
I go
I see
I don't know
Whether I was right or not
I did the right thing or not

Again the same conflict arises: not knowing the right way to raise the children and coping by staying busy, but anxiety returning when the solution she finds does not fulfil or provide a sense of security in her maternal ways.

Yasmin is in a quandary: either she protects her son, not allowing him to develop an independent identity, differentiated from hers, and leaving him vulnerable and insufficiently strengthened against life's toughness, or she releases him, voluntarily hands him over to the system, and in this way endangers him. Typically, this conflict raises anxiety and guilt in Yasmin, especially where anything happening to her child is concerned. It seems to have no real solution—a kind of zero-sum game, recurring in one or another version in many of the mothers.

Often a display of intense activity and ability constitutes a defence mechanism of "acting out" in the face of a sense of helplessness so great and threatening within that the individual cannot contain or express it. The self-confidence that Yasmin shows protects her from her internal truth of getting so lost in these debilitating sensations and anxiety that she would otherwise be paralysed. As Nietzsche writes in his first book, *The Birth of Tragedy* (1872): "Knowledge kills action, for in order to act we require the veil of illusion." Activity strengthens an emotional world that could shatter at any moment.

People like Yasmin sometimes stay more helpless than people capable of sharing these feelings.

As recruitment approaches

In the year prior to recruitment, as sons approach seventeen or eighteen, loss anxiety and helplessness among all the mothers appeared at high intensity, although in different ways. Their efforts were directed at delaying the coerced separation from the son. All of them talked about how, when the son was sixteen and the first recruitment notice arrived, their anxiety turned into real fear—as Lapid noted:

> "As soon as the first call-up paper arrived, Leah stuck it on the fridge, and everything changed with her . . . constantly crying and fearful, 'I don't want him to be a combatant.'"

The mothers tried to control the passing of time through detailed enumeration of the time frames still remaining before their sons' recruitment. This adoption of illusion concerning their ability to stop time serves the mothers in distancing the trauma.

Halting time

A disparity exists between the sense of motherhood time and external time, which moves forward consistently. It seems that, as enlistment approaches, the mothers focus on "the dimension of time" with increasing intensity, in an unconscious attempt to subordinate "external time" and even to suppress "internal time", which nonetheless acknowledges that the son is growing up—a wish that the years stand still in order to halt the encroaching danger. Additionally, it seems that this thought enfolds historical traumatic content, which seems to take on a life through the mothers' unconscious anxiety.

A similar use of the dimension of time is familiar from different historical periods and sources. In the battle fought by Joshua against the five Amorite kings in the thirteenth century BCE, Joshua commands the heavens: "Sun stand still in Givon, and the moon in the Valley of Ayalon . . . and the sun stood still in the heavens . . . and did not hurry to descend for a whole day. And there was none like that day, before or after it" (Joshua 10: 11–14). Halting time allows Joshua to achieve a sweeping victory.

Joshua's halted time became a cultural motif expressing the illusion that in order to fight death, it is possible to halt the machinations of the heavens, and therefore also time. In this way, for example, following the 1967 Six Day War, the song *Flowers in the Gun Barrel* by Dudu Barak was repeatedly played on the radio. It describes the silence of the morning after battle:

> The sun stands still between Gaza and Rafiah
> The moon whitens over the peaks of Mount Hermon
> Flowers in the gun-barrel, girls in the turret
> Back to the city the soldiers swarm.

The song goes on to describe an excited young girl who puts a flower in a soldier's lapel and ends with the hope that he who the day before was hurt or bereft would know no more war.

In 2002, Barak wrote another song with the same title. The song relates to the promise of peace "given to the current generation" and represented by the words of the earlier song. He returns to the same chorus of "The sun stands . . .". A woman expresses her wish to halt time in order to halt life in the shadow of war. The song also explains that the son did not know that the father went to bring peace. The Valley of Ayalon is mentioned as the place where the son is dreaming of the day fighting stops and breathing starts. Like a silken thread connecting past to present, the line from Joshua's wartime repeats itself here too.

Several historical events have occurred in the Valley of Ayalon since Joshua's time. In particular, in 1948, the Latrun area was considered a central axis that needed to be taken by the young Israel: it included the main road to Jerusalem and was the location of the famous convoys in and out of Jerusalem during the War of Independence. Three attempts were made to secure this area, and one of the most famous narratives of these battles involves Holocaust refugees being taken straight from the boats that brought them to Israel and being sent to fight in Latrun, where many were killed.

The precise repetition of the Biblical phraseology in the song also seeks to halt time in the context of longing for a cessation of all current wars, dreaming of peace.

The thousands of years of wars in the same place, with the added element of refugees who survived the Holocaust but died in war in that same location, gives rise, even if unconsciously, to the maternal fear that this is a destiny from which no single mother can save her son unless she applies the impossible technique used at the start of the historical chain, by halting the movement of sun and moon, and thereby the passage of time. As Becca said with such longing in her voice: "I want to send that year away."

Indeed, as well as behaving towards the sons as though they haven't grown up, and beyond the many verbal expressions indicating the attempt to halt time, the mothers have unconsciously activated an additional unrealistic perception of time by splitting their awareness of existential reality into *two units of time*: one up to recruitment, during which time they try to shape a world of only good (detailed below); the second, the son's actual period of military service, over which they have no control.

Leah tries to cope through magical thinking:

> "It's naïve but the thought accompanied me from birth . . . that in another month and half . . . there won't be any more war . . . and

> there are two months left . . . maybe there's more time. This is the first time I'm waiting for July *not* to come. And I so want to believe in it."

Becca also feels that the rhythm of time has changed and become too fast:

> "From high school on, the years go by fast . . . for three years I've had these fears . . . he wants to go to a fighters' unit, to elite commandos . . ."

Becca tried to convince her son to study for an additional year prior to recruitment—an attempt to intervene with the dimension of time—but his response was, "Enough, Imma, I can't sit on that chair any more."

Uncertainty and conflict

At this stage, a sense of heavy emotional stress on the mothers permeated the interviews, and separation from their sons took on the shadow of death. It seems that *lack of knowledge* about the brigade or unit to which their sons were to be recruited reinforces these feelings; as Becca said:

> "I don't know what to expect on enlistment day. He doesn't know where he's going either . . . what the conditions might be?"

The fact that a son can realize his own wish to serve in an elite unit, in opposition to his mother's wish, causes some mothers to experience their sons' choices of combat units as an act directed against them. Becca completely ignores the fact that her son is a young man facing a fateful decision in his life: she relates to his wishes as "the silliness" of a little boy aimed against her:

> "My son says, 'I want to shoulder the weapon and contribute to my country.' That's how they all are, they think they have to fight . . . I told him, 'Let's see what you have to say after three years . . . you can also serve close to home, and still contribute to the country.' So he says to me, 'I want to go through this the tough way!' He needs to choose . . . and he comes up with this rubbish. 'I want to be in undercover operations, or 669 Airborne Rescue.' 'Where did you get all this from?' I said to him, 'Take a bullet and shoot it in my temple right now! What sort of three years is that?' But he said, 'I don't want to be a desk soldier . . .' How silly!"

The feeling of "sitting shivah"

Among parents whose sons were about to be recruited, an atmosphere of *shivah*[8] was predominant. This is a time of mourning in which the mourners stay at home and are comforted by visits from family and friends, who cater to their every need. The parents interviewed conveyed the feeling that the worst thing of all had happened: they were in a kind of para–post-trauma awareness.

Dina and Becca, both of them highly emotional, tried to maintain restraint. Often the oppressive feeling came through more strongly from the silences and lowered eyes. Towards the end of her interview, Dina added:

> "I don't know if . . . I told . . . a thousand times . . . I imagine the moment . . . when we're informed . . . many, many times . . . I didn't bring it up here because it's so hard . . . I wanted to talk about it, but it's so hard for me to say this to myself . . ."

She rested her head on the table.

Leah, who didn't try to hide the weighty sense of mourning that filled her, said in a choking voice and in tears how a trip her son went on with the youth movement demonstrated the upcoming military service:

> "He was in the Scouts for three weeks, and I heard the song . . . *There's No Love Like a Mother's Love*, about a mother who made jam for her soldier son, and I remembered that weekend with him . . . and I really cried, out of longing . . . all those words touched my heart. It's the song that makes me totally emotional, and I cry and it hurts me and I'm hysterical . . . and I remember that young guy who was my kids' babysitter and was killed four years ago . . ."

She continued to describe the song, and I had tears in my eyes in the face of her pain and of my own longing and worry over Ari, my soldier son, who had recently begun his military service and came home only infrequently.

Sarit,[9] whose son was also pre-recruitment, took me to her son's room and showed me his things, in the way bereaved parents do. Her words also hovered around a song, *Lullaby*, which describes a mother who nicknames her son "Mother's little soldier" and promises the child that "Mother will protect you . . . and turn on the light when the war nightmares come." The world, and time, stop for her when her son is recruited.

Helplessness

Prior to recruitment, loss anxiety turns fear into the sense of real threat, which is contrary to the mothers' wishes and the emotional development process of the entire family. They are helpless when faced with this process, with very marginal control, as Dina describes:

> "Always . . . you hear the news and I see what happens to friends whose sons were recruited. My son will soon go into the army . . . I'm constantly wondering how I'll function . . . I'm so worried . . . if once a day I'll know where he is, then maybe I can get through it. I'm sure I'm going to go crazy during those three years . . . I won't be able to function . . . I see what my friends go through . . . life focuses completely on that, ups and downs in my mood . . . I don't see myself during those three years going for a week, say, overseas."

She then shared her concern over the change in the fabric of the family:

> "Now the sons want to come home, but how will things be later on . . . when they're in the army . . . I want it to go on like this . . . that they'll want to come . . . what will happen if he doesn't???"

Odelia also anticipated that she would feel helpless when her son does military service. Her fears are not experiences but manifest through somatization:

> "I repress thoughts about their recruitment, otherwise I get stomach pain because of it . . . it can't be coped with. The army is an intermediate point that I can't even think . . . imagine how to cope with . . . I'll keep some pills for that."

Behavioural patterns in Israeli mothers of sons

It is natural that such powerful feelings manifest in maternal behavioural patterns. And indeed, the mothers interviewed described a range of behaviours aimed at sabotaging, sometimes openly, sometimes covertly, processes of masculine identity consolidation in their sons—an identity that in Israel parallels the commando identity. This identity, perceived as superior to other identities, can only be attained through combat service. Its traits include: a muscular body marked, among other things, by wounds, even if minor; control over thoughts and emotions; control of weaponry and technology; toughness in the sense of emotional and physical robustness expressed through willingness to do tough, dirty work without hesitation and without showing disgust or laziness; overt competitiveness and ambition; a sense of adventure in life-threatening action; externalization of emotion and manifestation in situations that require self-sacrifice; a uniqueness that manifests through a "brothers-in-arms" confraternity; and exclusion of women from this male territory, on the one hand, while glorifying masculinity and all its components, on the other (Ben-Ari & Levy-Schreiber, 2000; Sasson-Levy, 2006).

It seems that the mothers intuitively knew what the masculine combat identity characteristics were—particularly the last, which excludes them. Through their maternal patterns they tried to fight the development process the very purpose of which is identity shaping. As Odelia said: "Recruitment of boys is a very central theme throughout the time they're being raised . . . whether consciously or unconsciously." The mothers' comments sketched a collage of interwoven parts that create a picture of "a secret mother-plan" for "how to raise wimpy sons without them knowing who did that to them".[10]

It was almost as though there had been an advance educational strategy, from pregnancy up until recruitment, sometimes conscious and sometimes unconscious: *to control* the process of the son's growing up in order to preserve him as a little child, shaping his character with as few masculine combat traits as possible while encouraging the feminine side and ignoring the sons' sexual development; and *to inhibit* the process of the son's separation from his mother, with the goal of trying to fight boys' natural tendency to continue into becoming combat soldiers.

The secret mother-plan

Computers, intelligence, and excellent musicians

A young male with good physical attributes is recruited into combat units and bestowed high social status compared to a non-combatant soldier called, in military slang, a "jobnik". For a son not to be a commando but also not a jobnik, which carries the slang connotation of "laflaf",[11] the mothers found a solution: to direct their future soldiers towards computers and/or the intelligence industry, neither of which hold danger to their lives yet still carry very high status on the masculine combat image scale since such units take only those with unique intellectual and/or educational levels, even if they are otherwise suited to a combat unit. As Galya said of her son, who would soon be entering school: "Let him go to Intelligence, or Computers, that's great. I don't want him to be a jobnik and feel worthless . . . let him do something respectable, help and contribute, without contributing his body."

The possibility of pressuring sons to excel in Arabic and computer sciences seemed to the mothers a successful solution to get their sons chosen for these units. This is clear from Galya's statement about her two small sons, one about to enter school the other just three years old: "I'll direct them both towards the Arab language track, so they can get into Intelligence rather than commando units . . . but maybe I'll only be able to influence one of them . . . they're both sensitive, but Roi more so than Itamar, so it's better if I influence Roi to go to Intelligence."

Ella explained that her difficulty was not the actual separation from her son; as proof she said that she prefers her son to study abroad, but guessed he would refuse and would want to enlist: "Let him go into the world, even to India or the Amazon jungle, for three years. At least let him gain something from it. I feel that it's less dangerous and has some value for him." Since this possibility is not realistic, she calms herself, saying "I constantly imagine that I can convince him to go into computers in the army, and then at least I'll sleep sound at night." The future anxiety over a son's life causes the mother to pressure him into developing in a way that responds to her needs rather than his as a separate individual with his own emotional world. Odelia, whose children were older, described how the plan is implemented in practical terms: "The only pressure I put on my oldest son is that he has to excel in Arabic. He laughs at me and knows I don't care about his other grades and that when he says, 'Imma, I got 100 in Arabic', I'm so proud. 'Carry on like that' . . . and he'll go into Intelligence, and that's a much safer feeling. He'd be bringing me this like a gift."

Yasmin and Yitzhak found another way out of the "decree"—serving as an accomplished musician or receiving an exemption on the basis of being a conscientious objector. Because the latter was contrary to the family values, they sent their children to a high school that educates towards such values, as Yitzhak explained: "We put them in a school where there's not even one soldier . . . the number of war fallen in that school is one." And Yasmin chimed in after him: "People who are all going to excel as musicians or are personal examples and don't enlist in the army."

In this way, through splitting (Klein, 1946), bringing the conflict out of the real of the intra-personal and projecting it onto that of the school's interpersonal realm, Yasmin does not have to contain the conflict within herself. She can allow her sons to receive these messages through the school's makeup and then express her opposition to them.

Odelia stated this quite clearly: "He loves to play all day, so I hope he'll go to an arts school, and they'll infuse a message of not going into the army . . . then it'd be his decision . . ."

Obliterating masculine traits and encouraging the feminine

The mothers battled primarily against masculine traits that belong to the "axis of control", exposing the ability to restrain and activate power on personal tendencies, needs, wishes, and emotions while encouraging traits like sensitivity and an artistic inclination which are opposite to strong, whole masculinity. Odelia demonstrated how she does this:

> "I developed a pattern with them where they can say anything they feel, even if we don't have an answer for it. I answer, 'You're right, that's very frightening . . . I don't think it's really going to happen . . . but it is very frightening.' And it seems this has been enough for them."

It would seem that Odelia is consciously driven by a wish to calm her sons' fears, but in fact she heightens them by validating fears without teaching how to regulate them. The outcome of this showed shortly afterwards, when her fears transferred to her sons, who said to her, "I don't want to go into the army. I don't want to die."

Hedy, whose older son was about to start school, said that she adopted an original strategy: to raise her sons as cowards, in order to direct them towards a non-combat track:

> "Amir said to me, 'Imma, a motorbike's dangerous, right?' I said, 'Oh, wow, and how. Of course it is.' Then I asked, 'What could happen if you're driving a motorbike?' and I added, '. . . and if you get hit . . .' Already at this stage, when he's young . . . get him afraid . . . I don't want them to be heroes. You see how much influence the army has! From the moment he started crawling, I got wariness into him. I don't want him to be too brave and go for overly frightening things. Yes, let him know what fear is! Even when he climbs a tree, I frighten him: 'Look how high it is, you can fall, and that will hurt . . . ' He doesn't have to be the one who jumps into the fire as though there's no tomorrow . . . I want him to think a bit before he does something . . . He doesn't have to be a great hero in the army. I don't want heroes."

The conflict with the longing to raise the ideal man of their imagination is given voice by Sara:

> "It's complex. On the one hand, you encourage him to let the tears flow, on the other, to hold them back. The message on the one hand is 'you need to be a man', on the other, be exactly the opposite."

In a bracing conflict of this nature, medical complications such as asthma or ADD, which can lower the son's military ranking and possibly make him unsuited for combat roles, are received by some mothers with relief and even seen as a blessing.

Limiting boys' war-game play

Studies that explored the correlation between watching or playing computer/video games containing violence, and violent behaviour among children and youths, offer contradictory findings.[12] The mothers, however, are taking no chances. As part of their maternal strategy for raising sons who will not be drawn into masculine combat behaviours, Naomi, Galya, and Hedy spoke out against every game that links, even associatively, with war. Naomi, pregnant, is not going to allow her son, as yet unborn, to play violent computer games, and was horrified on imagining all the aggressive energy. She declared early on that if her husband wants to take their three-year-old son to play football, she'll restrain that. My wondering what is wrong with playing football with Abba[13] was clarified later, when she shared that the only thing he'll have in his head is "football and cars . . . and then he'll go to the army".

Galya and Hedy said that when they were pregnant, they planned to prevent their sons from bringing games with anything like weapons into the house. When their boys were small, they initially forbade them to play any kind of violent game, but in the end they gave in to their sons over this prohibition, though with a sense of growing regret.

In the mothers' eyes, the father represents the masculine figure and is therefore responsible for what will happen. As such, part of their plan seems to be to strike out against the fathers' masculinity. The fathers cooperate with this situation unconsciously, which causes tensions in the couples' relationship (discussed further on).

Mothers spying on sons

It is important to emphasize again that though the mothers make open statements, they do not live the content openly in their daily lives, not even relative to themselves—precisely why the anxiety manifests unconsciously in their maternal patterns.

They tried, for example, to shape relationships of lack of separation with their sons, leaving no room for their privacy. Becca was angry when her almost eighteen-year-old son would not tell her whether he uses contraception. Dina complained that her sons do not share their lives with her even though she tries to get them to talk, because for her words are a communication tool. David, her husband, hearing this, noted with a loving smile that when school staff said parents should know where their children are, he thought that there isn't a moment when she doesn't know where they are. "If there is such a moment, she's already tense, starts phoning around to friends." Dina didn't deny this and even added how she found ways to spy on her sons, especially the one about to join the army:

> "I want to know what's happening with them after school. I badger them and ask direct questions. If I don't get an answer, I'll learn about it some other way, from mothers of their friends . . . from school . . . and I listen to his conversations with friends . . . I don't want to be disconnected from what's going on with them, so as not to be left . . . unprepared . . . so they won't be a big riddle. Sometimes I succeed, sometimes less. My oldest son, especially, is very withdrawn. He really doesn't tell us anything . . ."

It would appear that having experienced his mother's penetration of his space in a threatening manner, the son needs to close his reactions down almost completely. That is very difficult for Dina, and she understands that she overdoes it and therefore must respect her sons' boundaries. We might presume that this would lead Dina to letting go a little, but her anxiety causes her to try even harder. She talks to them about all her feelings, without deselecting the unsuitable from the overall, and so once again breaches the boundaries that her sons set.

Leah, whose firstborn was also about to be recruited, viewed this behaviour as legitimate: "I go into his room. *Without him knowing, of course*. To all the boys', but in recent years, more to Elhanan's . . . and check on his letters . . ."

Since his nursery school days and up to his finishing secondary school, Leah has acted in secret. She manages his life behind his back in order to prevent him opposing her: "Why argue with him?" she explains, then carries on in a completely self-satisfied tone: "I need to know every detail of his life, and Elhanan's friends tell me everything, even things that Elhanan has no idea I know . . . all kinds of things . . ."

When her husband, Lapid, expresses his opposition to her actions, she's not fazed at all; without any sense of conflict, she states that she's "she's not prying" but she "just needs to be up to speed". As proof of this, she details her son's primary characteristics and sums up: "Look, Elhanan's got his own thing going. But he came out *the way I wanted my son to be.*"

Through her behaviour, Leah had invaded the innermost workings of her son's psyche, making it harder for him to develop his own unique personality and for them both to develop the space for a mature relationship.

It is precisely through "maternal protection" that the sons pick up on their mothers' uncontained anxiety. Odelia's son is developing according to her expectations and excelling in Arabic, Sara's son lacks social skills, Dina's son is closed and withdrawn, and Leah's son has become a placating child based on a model predetermined for him by his mother.

Happiness, pleasure, and avoidance of conflict and boundaries: leading values in "Demeter's World"

I label the world the mothers are trying to create for their sons "Demeter's World". The Greek goddess Demeter, "the one who just gave birth", symbolizes motherhood and bestows crops and fruit. While in mourning over the kidnapping by Hades of her daughter Persephone, she became nursemaid to Demophon, a boy she wished to raise as an immortal. To achieve this, she never fed him human foods or allowed him to drink milk. Instead, she oiled his flesh, fed him the food of gods, allowed him to breathe her deific breath, and at night placed him in a burning fireplace. Demophon grew up wonderfully, but his human mother saw the child in the fire and thought he was being harmed. In response, Demeter drew him out of the fire, shouting angrily that ignorant humans are blind to their fate! She would have prevented Demophon from growing old, from death, and given him greatness, but now he would be like any other human (Shabtai, 2000, p. 20). The mother's voice, in shades and tones, repeatedly says: "He should just be happy."

Like Demeter, out of fear and guilt that they have no control "over the deaths of soldiers", Ruth, Sara, Galya, Odelia, and others try to build an "only good" world for their sons. Their decisions are goal-driven: for them and their sons to live happily and enjoy every moment of life.

This approach causes mothers to avoid expecting their sons to be achievers. Enveloping their behaviours in ideology, they exalt subjects or professions that require no effort to achieve, while foregoing the expectation of seeing their sons in professions that require education. As Galya explains: "We're here now, so it's preferable to take advantage of the moment." Or, as Ruth said, "A lot of adults have lost that basic *joie de vivre* that connects to the world of childhood . . . that's why it's important to see the half-full, to enjoy the small things, like gathering experiences, travelling, . . ."

Galya explained further:

> "All I want is that *things are good for him.* That he has friends, that he finds a girlfriend, that he marries her, and that . . . he finds work *that he loves.* It really doesn't matter to me what that work is. I met a nice guy, an older man, *full of joie de vivre* . . . and for the past fifteen years, he's been a courier. And he's such a wonderful man . . . *happy with his lot in life.* I don't care if my kids are like that, *if that's what they want, then they should just be happy with their lot. It's ok.* I don't have any goals that I want to reach. I don't expect a doctor, lawyer, or hi-techer, really I don't . . . it's not important to me."

She raised her right shoulder, then rested her head on it, in distress. If we understand that it is, in fact, important to her that her sons should become physicians, attorneys, and the like, but she is willing to forego all that for the sake of them not experiencing difficulty during their childhood—that is, if we assume that through her words she is using the negation defence mechanism that allows her to express verbal content while deselecting the hard emotional content by negating it—then we can further understand that Galya is coping with a tough conflict, one characteristic of the other mothers as well.

Of course, in Demeter's "only-good" world, the child has no separate boundaries. Even the air that the child breathes is her air. Indeed, boundaries are perceived by a large number of mothers as disruptive to creating the optimal, enjoyable life conditions for their sons. Ruth adopted an approach that life is a kind of game: everyone can decide for themselves to what extent to play by its rules. Therefore, she structured a world based on her rules for them, where she waives any demand that does not cause pleasure—including summertime tasks set by the school, which she considered a waste of their holiday. In this way, she restores the *sense of control* over her sons' destiny to herself, as though she successfully creates for them a world safe from all harm.

Even mothers like Hedy, Odelia, and Yasmin, who are aware of the need to fix boundaries, noted, while displaying a sense of conflict, that they easily waive demands on their sons to fulfil tasks that are not enjoyable, surrender to the sons in states of conflict, and do not feel good for standing their ground.

Conflictual situations arouse a sense of pain and sometimes also of isolation, but they allow children to familiarize themselves with, express, and develop their abilities as they consolidate their identity and independence. Parents' attitudes that constantly provide children with assistance convey a message that they lack the strength to cope independently, leaving them constantly "hanging", reliant on parents who help without allowing the child to undergo this important coping process.

For the son not to want to leave the Demetrian world, it must be infused with harmony and pleasure, and the best source of both is the mother. As Ella said:

> "So he won't be alone, so he'll always know that he can depend on me . . . that he's being related to, that he's being listened to, and that it's ensured he understands. So that he's connected, so he doesn't feel out of place . . ."

Another way to structure the Demetrian world is to avoid anger. For Ruth, the goal is to have children never encounter anger in the world. Ella didn't want to find herself in the morning persuading him to go to school. Yasmin turned the perception into an ideology:

> "If I'm really angry, what example of a mother do they grow up with? A mother who screams, a mother who's angry, a mother who gets infuriated???"

This, even though on other occasions she described, quite happily, how she argues with her daughters. Ruth also structured an ideology from her perception:

> "Knowing that they'll go to the army is hard for me. Whenever Rafael and I talk about this, he says, 'It doesn't matter how long you live, what matters is the quality . . .' We want to build a kind of greenhouse, to protect the kids . . . from the world. Maybe it's also linked to the education we think they should get."

Sara's outlook was uniquely her own:

> "I reached the conclusion that we're in this world for a particular purpose . . . I believe in reincarnation . . . and that we have a destiny . . . I do everything I can *to give him . . . everything in life that I can. To structure a different world for him,* but some things aren't dependent on me. So . . . it calms me to some extent. It's really hard for me to

let my sons go . . . I said to myself that as a mother my role is to support them. . . . When it was necessary, I went at the headmistress: 'If you don't let my son go on the field trip, I'm taking this to the education administration.'"

It seems, however, that deep in their hearts the mothers know that this is not the way to raise a son to realize his capabilities, and they are concerned. Sara demonstrated the damage she knows she's causing her son and her anxiety about his future ability to function in the army:

> "My son doesn't really function at school. I asked, 'What do you do in class?' He said to me, 'I count the number of times the teacher yells.' . . . Now I'm worried. He's constantly watching TV. I hope he'll come out of it over time. He doesn't have friends . . . hosting friends means making an effort, and he doesn't feel like it. It's sad . . . painful; I convince myself that as a mother I did what I could . . . he's a sensitive kid . . . wherever he goes, it'll be hard for him. In two years, he goes to secondary school . . . and then to the army. See, the thing that's constantly there in my mind is the army."

Sara's behaviour embodies contradictory messages. On the one hand, she tried to develop social tendencies in her son that would help him cope during his military service, but her actual intervention in his social life did not allow him to do so. In this way, she inhibited separation, development of independence, and the process that would allow him to adopt the masculine commando image that she experiences as endangering her life.

An unexpressed emotional conflict can manifest in somatic symptoms, where the physical ailment is the most common substitute for neurosis (Freud, 1895). Indeed, the mothers' emotional stress is projected on to physical symptoms in their children and in the mothers themselves. Galya talked about how one of her sons did not speak until he was three years old, another constantly blinked, a third experienced harsh pains in his leg, and there was a period when the sons clung to Galya in a way that made things really tough for her. Since she entered into an emotional whirlwind each time, which included comprehensive physical check-ups that revealed that the symptoms had no physiological source, it could be that the psychic content of anxiety over their lives was being converted into physical symptoms that manifest parallel content (Freud, 1895). This offered her a solution that enabled her to evade feeling the conflict, both because the anxiety found an alternative avenue for manifestation, and because sons with medical issues are unsuitable for combat service. Odelia expressed this reality when she showed happiness that one of her sons suffered from ADD, which, she hoped, would mean he would not be recruited as a combatant.

Moving to "Act II" before the sons' recruitment

When the time for recruitment arrives, the mothers discover that their plans have not succeeded, that they cannot truly control their sons' destinies. The suddenness of this transition is emphasized by the fact that once a son receives his first call-up papers, he becomes, in legal language, "the IDF's asset". He is called for various selection processes, ending with the IDF's decision, slotting him into a specific brigade. He cannot leave the country without authorization from the army, and he could be penalized by law if he fails to appear at the recruitment office on the appointed date.

Recruitment to elite commando units, which carries very high social status, is voluntary: the sons can themselves decide whether they wish to join. The mothers know this, so they focus their efforts on persuading their sons not to volunteer for these units—at the same time transitioning to "Act II": tactics that perpetuate the relationship between mother and young child, without taking into consideration the son's true age and his masculine focus. For example, Leah's husband said:

> "In our conversations the fear constantly surfaces, she repeats again and again that sentence, 'I don't want him to be a commando' . . . she'll get angry if I say this, but it's the truth: he had an internal matriculation test at the same time as a call-up for the paratroopers and *Duvdevan* [elite commando] capability trial days. She turned the world upside down to make me convince him to go to the exam, not the trial . . . anything to block this issue of . . . commando."

From the way the mothers describe their relationships with their sons, it would seem that their emotional and behavioural patterns *lead to not giving space, worry over their sons' physical and psychic well-being, and difficulty in allowing their sons to distance themselves from them.* Instead of easing off the growing son approaching recruitment, mothers try to reinforce their hold on him, even through coercion. Becca and Dina, both mothers of sons about to enlist, said they tried to convince their sons to study for an additional year. Becca added: "We told him, 'You'll get anything you want—a car . . . anything . . . the main thing is that you study for another year.'"

Boaz felt he needed to be precise: in a critical tone he said Becca would do anything, but the main thing is that the son would be close to home.

Dina understood that recruitment is no longer in her control; she tried to track her son's whereabouts and activities by mobile phone, but the son, feeling that his mother was controlling him via the phone, refused to accept this arrangement. Her husband said he was having none of it and gets mad when she calls his friends.

Anna Freud emphasized that one of the typical processes of adolescence is the acceleration in sexual urges and fantasies. The adolescents absorb their parents' sexuality more maturely, feel a sense of internal threat, and display embarrassment when facing the force of these new emotions. As a result, adolescents find it difficult to maintain the relationship with their parents, especially with the parent of the opposite sex. This is an age when it is natural for adolescents to distance themselves from parents as they seek other figures of identification and emulation and transmute the love kept only for the mother to a couple relationship that is outside the family. The entire process is meant to be gradual and suited to the personal needs and pace of the adolescents and their mothers.

Anna Freud (1936) pointed out that a process of libidinal detachment that is too rapid expresses a disorder in the developmental process and sabotages normally developing separateness. The compulsory recruitment to military service intervenes blatantly with the delicate developmental processes in the relationship with sons and constitutes a sudden detachment by the son from his mother. From the interviews, this does indeed appear to be the experience of the mothers, who feel a basic need to oppose their sons' maturity and detachment from them.

Covert value-based conflicts arising parallel to the desire to navigate sons into a decision not to become commandos

It is highly complex for a mother to raise childish, dependent sons in a country where military service is, first and foremost, an existential need, where the masculine identities of fathers and grandfathers are consolidated and values such as contributing to society, mutual involvement and responsibility, maintaining national existence, and more are realized.

Femininity develops through the unique relationship with fathers; therefore, the dimension of the mother's relationship to the father's masculine values and identity, and the woman's primal attraction to the commando soldier husband, all affect the mother's femininity and further complicate things. Additionally, another level of the mother exists—the woman who bears the cultural baggage of the mythical Israeli Jew, from which she has shaped her moral and social value system. It is understandable that when these layers pull in opposite directions, the mother finds herself in a deeply conflictual emotional maelstrom, a great part of it in the unconscious, without the ability to find a single solution that would address the contradictory internal tugging.

Unlike the basic conflict shared by all mothers between the wish to allow the son to develop a separate independent identity and the wish to raise him in safety and protect his life, when it comes to expressing conflict in the context of others, each mother copes with her own typical content.

Hedy, nearing the end of pregnancy with a male fetus and already with two young boys, was adamantly opposed to her sons' future military service. Thinking about the time until they were to be recruited, she said:

> "It won't be so pleasant for me to slowly lodge in their minds that they shouldn't be combat soldiers . . . because I know someone has to enlist and fight. I think it won't be so nice for me to tell them to go to this or go to that. But I wouldn't want them to go for commando . . . especially if there's a war in Lebanon, or some other war."

She paused, then said decisively:

> "When I think about it, I see that in my everyday life I navigate them towards a lifestyle where they won't be commandos. I really don't want them to be commandos."

Her understanding of the situation confronted her with an additional value-based contradiction: even though she said that she finds *freedom of choice* to be a very important educational principle, she found herself fearfully stating that when they're eighteen, she'll have to let her sons choose which brigade they want to serve in. And then another course of action occurred to her:

> "If they ask me questions, I think I'll . . . show opposition: yes, he wants to be a paratrooper, but I'll suggest maybe it's worth him being something else."

The image of her sons as paratroopers matches her own father's values as a paratrooper in the 1967 Six Day War, on whose stories of heroism in military service she grew up. She said:

> "I wasn't raised that way. My father was a paratrooper, and I was so proud of that. It's really not pleasant for me to do the opposite . . . to educate him that way, even though inside myself . . . I prefer my son to be in the *Shekem*."[14]

Dina found herself in a different kind of conflict:

> "A commando son is scary, but there's also some kind of pride, because . . . it's important to me, and it wouldn't occur to me that . . . to tell him, to evade it . . . I internalized that it's admired . . . my neighbour's son's a pilot, or a commander, or someone really successful in the army, these are the admired guys. We look a lot less nicely on someone who shirks his duty. For example, David's cousin became ultra-Orthodox and didn't serve, so we really disdain him . . ."

Giving expression to the side of the conflict that identifies with the values of commando service brought feelings of guilt; Dina clarified how she tries to evade them:

> "I'm really wary of a situation where our son goes to a commando unit because we expect it, and he doesn't want to disappoint us. I found my own stupid solution: I just won't tell him which brigade to join . . . I'm afraid to say anything, because if I do . . . and something happens, then I'll eat my heart out later."

Galya and Gad tossed thoughts around the conflict between each other like a hot potato. Galya spoke very determinedly against her sons' future recruitment to commando units, but Gad said:

> "She's conflicted, because she says she doesn't want her sons to be commandos, but her reactions to the recent terror attacks are very strong, and militant. She says we should really give it to them . . ."

They argued until Galya settled the conflict inside herself:

> "I'm not militant . . . but there was a house where they constantly shot at us from . . . only two months later, they took that house

> down with a mortar. I said they should have reacted sooner, because people got hurt during those two months. I'm not saying we should go into a settled village . . . and that's . . ."

It seems that describing images of battle raised images in her mind of her sons taking part in such situations, together with feelings of guilt over her support for the militant approach. And just like that, in one go, Galya set her position concerning her sons: "They can also go to Intelligence or such things, they don't have to be a pilot that sends the . . ." Then she rested her hand on her belly, as though protecting the fetus inside: "They can go to research to develop the missile, they don't have to be the pilot that drops the missile."

To kiss and hug more, or less, because "they're going to the army"?

Occasionally the maternal conflicts are not on the surface. They arise, for example, from within Ella's somewhat oblique statements. Ella's son is about to enter school.

> "To set clear boundaries, in my view . . . not to scrimp on love, I . . . I don't kiss them less because they're going to the army, but when I tell them something, I mean it, and I try . . . I try to be consistent, sometimes it's not so pleasant for me, but I do try to be consistent."

We can understand the educational message in her statements, which are based on coherence in education. Perhaps when she says she has no intention of holding back in her love for her sons, that she doesn't kiss them any less because they'll go to the army, she is demonstrating her opposition to raising her sons according to the "control-axis" approach of educating to emotional restraint in view of their future recruitment (Sasson-Levy, 2006). However, observing her "I-Poem", where the first line becomes the title, reveals additional layers that Ella is perhaps less conscious of:

> I don't kiss—because they're going to the army
> When I say
> I mean
> I try
> I try
> I try

It seems that Ella perhaps feels she succeeds only in "trying" to be consistent. Going back to the first line, "*To set clear boundaries,* in my view, not to *scrimp on love* . . . I don't *kiss them less because they're going to the army*"—if we remove the negation words—based on our understanding, as Freud (1925) explained, that it allows verbal expression of harsh emotions while avoiding their threatening emotional content—we arrive at the following statement: *to set clear boundaries, to scrimp on love, to kiss less, because they're going to the army.* The existence of conflict begins to reveal itself.

This excerpt can be understood in various ways. Starting at the simplest level: does knowing of her sons' recruitment cause Ella to want to kiss them a lot and to love them without limits, which contradicts her understanding that boundaries are important in educating children? Or, conversely, is the knowledge that her sons "will go" to the army, which accompanies Ella's mothering—where her use of "go" alludes to their going from her and hence separating from her—cause Ella to withhold her love from them by kissing them less? If so, what is the source driving this action? Is it anger over a future time when they will leave her? Perhaps anger over the advance knowledge of the end outcome, when they will join the "masculine combat party"? Or is she trying to control her great love for her sons, and her wish to kiss them a lot, from a wish for self-protection against the most terrible fear of all—which she expressed throughout the interview—that her sons might go from her into a world where they will be killed in the army? Could it be that Ella thinks that a tougher attitude will prepare them better for what awaits them in the army?

A hint of what this all means to Ella can be found at the end of the interview, when she says:

> "The issue of the army came up only in me. It's impossible to ignore it as a very big transition in the life of this son of mine, and the sentence 'he'll go to the army' constantly plays in my mind. It's not that it drives me nuts, but it's always there somewhere . . . And because of it there are things I do in my daily life, and especially things I'm more meticulous about. I justify my action in the context of 'how will it be in the army' . . . maybe by being aware of it, we do things differently."

Although Ella's statements shed light on her point of view, with the limited research tool of one interview and the point in time when it was conducted, there is no way of knowing with absolute certainty which understanding of the conflict's significance is correct. It is only possible to take note of the emotional forcefulness and complexity in the mother as a result of the knowledge of her sons' future recruitment, which is intertwined with, and complicates, her mothering at the emotional, conceptual, and practical levels.

Educating towards emotional expression or aggression?

Sara shared the confusion in which she finds herself:

> "We raise them here to violence. The question is, how to raise them? We're supposed to raise them not to get angry, not to hit, but they encounter violence everywhere. They need to be aware and know how to use force and their abilities. It . . . makes it hard for me. On the one hand, the child needs to be taught to control his force, to retaliate. On the other, we don't want him to use his power. But that's the reality where we live . . . if he cries, then on the one hand my message is to let the tears out, on the other to hold back? . . . On the one hand you need to be a man, on the other you want . . . that if he's hurting, he can say so and cry."

I asked what she did, how she behaved. Distressed, she continued:

> "That's . . . always a dilemma. You say to him, 'Stop crying' and then immediately continue, 'Cry, cry.' See? It seems to me that I'm conveying a dual message . . . no???"

Galya—pregnant with a son—was also busy with the issue of messages conveyed around violence; she recounted a conversation she had with her four-year-old son: "He asked me really wonderful questions for a four-year-old." Then suddenly, a disconnected statement: "Yes, I raise him to have tolerance."

And again, as though without connection, she continues:

> "He asked me if we take the Arabs we shoot at to hospital, or just let them die? I said they're taken to hospital. So he asked, 'Why? They'll just take a gun again and shoot . . .' That's an amazing question . . . it took me a few minutes to think, and then I said, 'They'll get better and then we'll punish them in prison for what they did.' And he accepted that . . ."

Then she suddenly raised her voice in anger against Gad, who had previously claimed she is militant:

> "I'm not militant. I don't say 'let's give it to them', so that he'll understand it's not all just about confrontation. That's part of educating . . . I'm trying to educate to humaneness and assertiveness, but I still don't want them going to the army . . . It's clear to me that if there's no choice, and you're being attacked and shot at, then at least the building where the shooting's coming from, or the olive grove, as terrible as it sounds, that they're hiding there and shooting at you and your people are being killed, so you need, with all the sorrow in it, to . . . uproot it. Yes, better to uproot it than have people killed . . . So I'm trying to teach him humaneness and assertiveness."

Is recruitment to the army looked at entirely negatively by the mothers, or are there also "a few good points" about it? By contrast to Leah, who utterly negated combat service for her son, Dina's and Becca's words echo values that side with recruitment. Dina said:

> "It's hard to think that recruitment is only bad, because it's really hard to educate towards that . . . it can't be that there are no positive points about the entire Israeli army . . . When it goes well, I heard that it 'organized, consolidated the kid' . . . that they're considered 'salt of the earth' and 'quality', the ones that took part and got things done. And later, in civilian life, they're given a lot of credit; I heard that for the position of warehouse manager they wanted only someone who'd been a commander in the military . . . Maybe that makes it easier for me, because if he doesn't serve, he'll bear the mark of Cain in Israeli society, he won't be accepted in certain places . . ."

The physical fitness that her son began developing as recruitment time approached was the only good point that Becca could find. She laughed tensely and said:

> "He paid money for combat fitness twice a week, came back from the 'stretchers trek' totally covered in dust . . . in order to be ready . . . At least he's keeping up his fitness, so I don't care that he trains . . . instead of playing football."

Signs of moving towards independence such as this are indications of the process of maturation and separateness in the son. Thus, despite failing in the maternal task of creating their sons' conditions of self-confidence, the mothers tried to comfort themselves by viewing some of the sons' activities as indicating that they did develop independent separate identities, which is also a way of measuring the mothers' success.

Patterns of "clutching behaviours" and "releasing behaviours"

Patterns of clutching behaviours towards sons

I wish to coin the term "clutching behaviours" to describe maternal behaviours aimed at resisting any process in which separation from the son would allow him to undergo the process of separation and consolidation of a separate identity (Chodorow, 1978). Balancing this out, I would term "releasing behaviours" behavioural patterns that allow the son to undergo processes of separation and separateness.

Recruitment day is determined by the military authorities, notwithstanding the son's readiness or maturity to separate from his parents or the parents' emotional readiness to allow this separation. In all interviews of mothers with sons close to recruitment, when they imagined the moment, their emotional dam broke, and they spoke of military service in powerful terms, the threat to their sons' lives becoming tangible. Their wish to *clutch* the son close to them collided with the need to let him go. *The feeling arising in me was one of a collective experience in a tribe that knows what is about to occur.*

The moment of recruitment, when mothers accompany their sons to the recruitment centre and their sons board the buses that take them away, drains the maternal anxiety that has accrued throughout the years of raising their son. From this point on, the mothers felt, the nature of their relationship with their sons would change. Orit Lavnin–Dgani (as quoted in Isachar, 2003), describes it this way:

> On the day that my son enlisted, it was as though my legs were severed. I barely got through that day, and for the next few months found it hard to get used to the feeling that they're erasing the child. . . .

I met with the three mothers shortly before their sons' actual recruitment day. They shared the same emotional difficulty, but their behavioural patterns and reactions varied.

Leah did not change the controlling pattern typical of her mothering, which ignored changing reality and drew her to fighting that reality; she resisted Lapid, who told her that she forbids her son various things, but that she should keep in mind that he will soon be a soldier.

Dina and David deliberated on how much responsibility they should give their firstborn, about to be recruited, over his studies, and how responsible they should continue to be. Dina felt that since her son was soon to be keeping guard over her, a kind of inversion of roles would occur that neutralizes her parental role, including her authority. Showing discomfort, she said:

> "It's hard to start behaving towards him . . . I'm starting to get used to the fact that in just . . . a few months he'll . . . need to take decisions alone . . . I don't know . . . maybe his recruitment makes it more tangible, really changes things. We relate to him more like an adult. He'll be going soon . . . to keep guard over me, so how can I tell him when to go to sleep . . ."

Sadness filled the room as she described feeling that these were the final moments in which she *clutches* her son. She used the word "slacken", as in slow down, decelerate; loosen; ease, make less intense. When *clutching* is experienced as protecting the child, slackening means abandoning this protective state.

All the mothers, irrelevant of their sons' ages, planned to give the sons a mobile phone, so that they could stay in close contact with them. When Hedy thought about future recruitment, she said: "I know that if my son's in the army, I'll be in a panic, everything will frighten me, already now it's clear to me, phone calls . . . and how, and how!"

Ruth—with three sons: one ready to start school, one aged three, and one less than a month old—also related to this issue.

> "When I think about the army, and the involvement of parents and the media, and mobile phones for children, I see that the army fights parental intervention, and I don't know how I'll behave. I'm sure it'll be really hard for me, because that really is a loss of control . . . it's as though it's not entirely in my hands . . ."

Ella, the second of whose three sons was about to start school, and whose oldest son was ten at the time of the interview, shared her fantasy that through the mobile phone she would give her son's commander instructions, and that the phone can correct, to some small extent, what the army ruins in the relationship between herself and her son:

> "They'll go into the army, and we'll have those same fears, and mothers will fight. I'm great with them having mobile phones nowadays, to stay in touch. I'm told that mothers phone and ask to speak to the commander . . . I really like that idea."

Dina's comments seemed to join in here:

> "When he gets to the army base, if he doesn't phone, at the least . . . once a day . . . but I don't believe he will do that. So I'll call him. If he's not accessible, I'll really get uptight."

Leah was not calmed by the thought of phone contact with her son; she said: "My friend Goldie said that she thought, before the army, that the moment he's recruited it'll be easier for her . . . which I don't believe, because I don't . . ."

Leah's husband Lapid interrupted: "I hope so, because I don't intend to spend every weekend at the base." Leah burst into laughter. Lapid laughed too, then looked at me when Leah added: "I will! I'll go!"

The feeding motif in the maternal relationship with sons in the army

When the mothers imagined the moment of meeting their recruited sons, either when he comes home from his base or when they visit him at the base, they described a recurring image of feeding their sons. Every Israeli is familiar with the image of parents coming on the Sabbath[15] to their sons' bases loaded with pots and pans and baked goods—as though the army lets everyone go hungry. The mothers orchestrate this most primal activity of feeding, typifying the relationship between the mother and her newborn, as Becca described:

> "Then the butterflies in my stomach are more . . . get stronger . . . it's really frightening . . . I'm sure if he doesn't come home on any particular Sabbath, we'll be out there on base with our pots of food."

Or, as Lavnin-Dgani (quoted in Isachar, 2003) describes, following her son's recruitment:

> "The questions you ask him—Did you eat? Drink? Are you dry? . . . You go backwards eighteen years with him: he's a baby again."

Beyond diminution of the son through the act of feeding, what is conveyed through the physical action—as in the process of assimilation—is a message containing the dimension of control. The mother will decide what goes into her son's mouth and how much: in this way she becomes "his master"—or, rather, "his mistress"—instead of the army, much like God saying to Ezekiel, "'Son of man . . . eat this roll and go speak to the House of Israel' . . . and I opened my mouth and he fed me this roll . . . and I ate it and it was like honey, sweet in my mouth" (Ezekiel 3: 1–3) or Freud (1939) who parallels this Biblical scenario to the Christian Mass in its maternal connotation, in which the son eating the food that the mother prepared with her own hands symbolizes assimilation of her body in his, and in this way the fantasy of total fusion is almost complete.

Patterns of "releasing behaviours" towards sons

It is important to present, parallel with mothers' voices resisting their sons' separateness, voices that accept the process of separation that sons need to undergo.

There were several spots where Odelia spoke with ambivalence but without panic:

> "It's been clear to me that I'm raising my sons to independence and to leave me . . . that I'll be left . . . It's impossible to be left by girls. But . . . sons need to go . . . I want to hold onto them, but I can't."

Her professional development helped create space between herself and her sons:

> "After I accepted this, and started developing my career, I began to enjoy my life. It's important for me to be satisfied with my professional life . . . The decisions I took in my career occurred . . . parallel to separating from my sons. It sounds very cruel, but . . ."

Odelia managed to function in both clutching behaviour and releasing behaviour patterns, an emotional functioning that requires the emotional ability to contain the conflict that accompanies motherhood:

> "When they were small, I was really close to them. I spent a lot of time with them . . . full-time . . . and separation from them was always difficult for me . . . so the army has an impact, and that's also positive, because the process of separation from sons is natural, and I couldn't have done it easily if I hadn't known that I must."

In their hearts, the mothers knew they could not change the fact of recruitment. Some began to think about how to prepare their sons for coping with the future. Some tried to integrate additional behaviours into their protective behaviours, as a way of readying the sons for coping with military service. These wishes often led to conflict.

We already encountered the maternal feeling that sending children to school is like sending them to the army. From this starting point,

Odelia felt that sending her sons to a school that is not too protective would prepare them better for military service.

> "After all, the world isn't a simple place, and we need to know how to cope. For me it was a really difficult issue . . . I'm ashamed to admit, but . . . there's this thought . . . that it's not good to continue protecting them . . . part of me is aware of this from a very young age, that I'm raising them and preparing them for the army . . . we do try to ready them and provide them with all the skills possible without harming their development, like learning another language, how to cope with conflict . . ."

Ella also raised her sons to independence in order for them to function in the army:

> "I try to develop his capabilities of independence as much as possible. Sometimes a bit to the extreme . . . I deliberate over whether that's right, and then I say, he needs to get there in the end . . . In the army they won't give him special consideration, won't speak to him in the most pleasant manner, and he'll need to take decisions he may not like. I have so many arguments with my oldest son: that life isn't always easy, that we do things not because we want to but because we need to. When I ask for assistance and he says 'Not now', I say: 'I need your help now, not when you feel like it.' . . . I'm also lovey-dovey with them, but I also have these really rough spots with them. It's because they need to go . . . into the army, into life, to develop their independence, to do things by themselves."

Towards the interview's end, Ella said:

> "It's constantly humming at the back of my mind, like a song: there's the army . . . that it won't be better or easier, and I carry on. Today the conversation linked the words and the melody for me. . . . Why be tough already now with the child? After all, there are a few years left. He's still so very young. It's interesting, the fact that I spoke about it, suddenly I stopped to think, and it allows me something new."

Overprotectiveness of sons

Of all the examples presented above, the pattern of overprotectiveness stands out, such as with Yasmin: she's constantly on guard, checking if they've done their homework, if they've practised their music; she knows where they are at every moment, advises and directs them.

The Israeli poet Ayin Hillel's poem "Yossi, My Successful Little Boy" is about a mother protective of her son in a way that does not match his age. The poem describes repeatedly how Yossi's mother sends him out to buy milk, and each time the child gets caught up instead in doing something else. The mother never becomes angry with him or confronts him over the outcome of his behaviour and, in an inverse reaction, calls him "my successful little boy". She comforts herself that the house is full of love, even though there is no milk or bread.

She does not allow herself to know that by overly protecting Yossi, she is raising him to be a non-functioning individual. Her relationship with her son, like the relationships of the mothers in this research, is characterized by fusion and the blurring of boundaries. She does not differentiate between her wishes and those of her son—a relationship pattern that typifies the period of pregnancy and early infancy (Winnicott, 1960). The mothers described a range of behaviours that seem to preserve or extend for as long as possible the experience of sons safe under their wings.

The mothers adopt an approach whereby good motherhood requires

> . . . unconditional love, which assumes that from a loved child, something unloved, harmful, or painful for those who love the child cannot emerge. . . . This approach is responsible for parents doing backward somersaults in their logic and emotions in order to not see or not be hurt by those things that their sane capabilities are unable to love . . . and we see its destructive outcomes in everyday life and read about them in newspapers. [Lewow, 2011]

We have seen how the mothers feel guilty over not being able to protect their sons from the encroaching threat to their lives, but perhaps another aspect rests within their covert acknowledgment of the damage inherent to their behaviours. As Becca said:

> "I have mixed feelings . . . I'm afraid he'll do his service in Tzrifin or the Kirya, 'doing the eight five'[16] and . . . he'll come home . . . and eat my heart out: 'It's all your fault . . . what kind of army am I doing, picking up crates, stacking papers. I don't want this, it's not suited to me.'"

Dina stared into her glass of tea and whispered:

> "Somehow all my kids came out . . . not too free . . . and I can understand it with a mother like this . . . I think it has to do with recruitment . . . they need to put a boundary between them and me, otherwise there won't be enough separation, they need to block me, because I'm very interested, and sometimes . . . break boundaries."

Unconscious developmental process

The roots of guilt feelings in an individual draw on deep unconscious sources, the system of patterns and values internalized by the individual—the superego (Freud, 1923).

According to Freud, for individuals to accept their sexual urges and develop the feeling of being alive and of belonging, even where they are not the centre of attention, they need to be allowed as children to feel loved and belonging—including when faced with the sexual intimacy between the child's parents into which the child is not invited. Freud (1915b) termed this dynamic, "primal phantasies". A later, significant emotional development, which Freud called "the Oedipus complex", begins in boys when they become aware that they have a sexual organ that girls lack. This awareness raises the anxiety that "father will castrate them, as he must have done to the girls as punishment for the attraction they feel towards their mother". This fantasy brings identity displacement from the mother to the father and is a necessary process for the successful transition from the close relationship with the mother to a three-way relationship: father, mother, and son. It is a stage that allows the son reaching adolescence to shift his strong love for his mother to another female partner. The dynamic resurfaces during the course of life. Freud emphasizes the importance of protecting the ego against castration anxiety. Since waiving the cathexis towards the oedipal object and its substitute by identifying with the parental authority, the core of the superego comes into being and allows the ability to take control over the course of life (Loewald, 2000).

If this stage is accompanied by difficult emotional experiences of rejection or, alternatively, overstimulation, the psyche will tend to repress the existence of the sexual aspect in the individual. The more violent and powerful the repression of the Oedipus complex, the more will a controlling and depressive superego develop. In other words, the sense of guilt is a kind of self-violence that the ego activates on the self, and it needs no rational source in external reality (Freud, 1923).

Although a girl undergoes a different development process, which may leave her loyalties with her mother, Freud attributed a less severe superego structure to woman. For the mothers interviewed, it might be that because they are unable to allow their sons to distance from them, the entire system finds difficulty in undergoing the oedipal processes, and the mothers are flooded by guilt, control, harsh self-judgement, and judgementalism towards the rest of the environment; they are therefore typified by expanded and particularly active superegos, as I detail further on.

Ogden (1989) defined guilt as a certain kind of pain that the individual carries over a period in reaction to a real or imagined injury caused to someone else the individual cares about. Individuals may try to correct what they feel guilty about, but doing so does not void what has been done, and they may therefore develop compensatory behaviour in future relationships over what has been done to others or themselves.

Since the mothers perceive the Israeli reality into which their sons are born as one that inherently contains a threat to their sons' lives, they try to create an opposite reality, in which they both compensate the sons for the injustice they feel has been done to them and address their own guilt feelings as mothers who have given birth to sons in such a reality.

"Splitting", one of the psychic defence mechanisms a person uses when it is too difficult to bear the emotions deriving from life's reality, is derived from the attempt to achieve a sense of security by separating what is in danger from what is not. In this emotional state, what might have turned into the sense of guilt is dissipated, such as through omnipotent fantasies of correction, where the injury to the other is refuted through the use of magical correction (Ogden, 1989). In this way, for example, by creating a protected world, the mothers try to build *a reality split from all evil* for their sons; every dangerous or frustrating thing is left outside that world, thereby distancing and repressing the sense of approaching threat brewing in their psyches, a feeling that accompanies and disrupts their mothering.

Mothering girls compared to mothering boys

Although this study is presented as relating to "the thoughts and feelings accompanying raising of children", in all the interviews the parents focused chiefly on the sons—especially on the son chosen for the study. As stated previously, the parents were unaware that they had been chosen because they had sons, nor that my interest was relative to a specific age group. When the mothers mentioned daughters,[17] it was usually to demonstrate the difference in their relationship with them compared to their relationship with sons, or to show differences in the personalities and behaviours of boys compared to girls.

A consistent picture began to form where, in contrast to their attitude towards sons, the mothers allowed their daughters greater space to develop a separate personal identity, and they viewed the daughters' independence as their personal achievement. Psychoanalytic studies and literature have not delved into the conscious and unconscious emotional processes undergone by women when they become mothers and during their motherhood, and the same applies to fathers (Palgi-Hecker, 2005; Sayers, 1991).

From the current study, it would appear that, in Israel, mothering boys is very different from mothering girls. It could be claimed that the difference derives from the fact that, compared to the separation from the mother inherent in adopting a masculine identity among boys, girls preserve the connection with the mother when developing their feminine identity (Block, 1973; Chodorow, 1978;[18] Gilligan, 1982). It would be logical to assume that, despite the difficulty, the mother at this stage would experience satisfaction from the very fact of succeeding in her maternal task to raise an independent son with a unique masculine identity. However, as we have seen, since separation from the son is identified with future military service, the mothers—apart from Odelia and Dina—filled their mothering with loss anxiety, feelings of helplessness, and guilt. Interviewees who were mothers only to sons described the experience of raising girls idealistically, and as being free from the emotional burden that they, as mothers, bore relative to their sons. Mothers of both boys and girls experienced mothering girls as one of space and joy, as Leah describes:

> "When my daughter Hadar was sixteen, she spent three weeks in Holland . . . I was so glad; but when Elhanan was seventeen, he spent three weeks on a scout trip, and my longing for him was pronounced, yet I love them the same. I don't understand . . . I don't love more but . . . I'd hear that song by Zehava Ben about her son . . . *There's No Love Like a Mother's Love,* and I'd cry."

Hedy— with two young sons, and pregnant with another—said that she wants a daughter, because a son ". . . is another child I have to send to the army . . . and I'm worried . . . On the other hand, with boys, I don't need to cope with the brouhaha of girls, so maybe it's easier."

But then her anxiety resurfaced: "But with boys, there's the worry later over the army . . . and it's different than with girls . . . No! It's harder with boys than with girls."

When Ella, who for most of the interview focused on her sons' future conscription, tried to imagine what it would be like to mother girls, she didn't think about the army. Her husband, Eitan, reminded her that girls serve for two years, but she answered: "Girls just waste their time in the army unless they have a chance to do a '*Ka'datz*'.[19] But we're very curious about what it's like to raise a girl."

Her easygoingness when reacting to military service for girls was particularly noticeable compared to her expressions of strong distress when discussing her sons' military futures.

Ruth, for whom raising sons is also rife with loss anxiety, said:

> "We've got sons. With girls there's a lot less real and existential anxiety. It's selfish that I want a daughter . . . The connection between a daughter and her mother is much freer, it's easier . . . not the same as a son and mother. That's something else altogether, talking with sons or talking with daughters . . . you can even talk with them about the Holocaust. With my sons it's 'yes', 'no', 'black', 'white'. With daughters it's different."

By using the Holocaust as an example, Ruth tried to demonstrate that closeness with a daughter is free from pain and anxiety to the extent that it is even possible to talk with her about events that inherently enfold traumatic separation through death.

Naomi, mother of a fourteen-year-old daughter and about to give birth to her first boy, shared her fantasy about mothers to daughters: "Motherhood of daughters is different in a very significant way . . . I don't know why. Maybe because it's easier for me with girls in general, it's clearer to me."

She detailed a string of worries over the life of her son, not yet born. When her husband wondered why she was so worried about a son, yet felt confident about her daughter, Naomi responded: "It really is a bit absurd, because I should be worrying more about a daughter."

A list of anxieties or strategic behaviours towards daughters paralleling those relative to boys could not be found. In fact, the opposite is true. Sara, Leah, Dina, Becca, and Yasmin described their daughters as independent, opinionated, and self-confident, compared to their weak sons, who require supervision, guidance, and orientation. These descriptions reflect the existence of a comfortable mother–daughter space in which they exist, and separateness and independence are allowed to develop parallel to the relationship, as described by Naomi:

> "I worry that maybe I'll be more critical of a son. Actually, there's anxiety over a son . . . I think that if my daughter has lice, ok, that arouses less anxiousness . . . it's clearer . . . I don't understand what's happening here . . . For me, boys are characterized by not being open, neither with themselves nor with their environment, so I think that maybe they're more fragile."

When referring to adolescent girls, Leah, Becca, and Sara went into issues typical of independent personality development while breaking conventions and boundaries. This topic did not surface in mothers talking about sons. Sara's anxiety focused on studying and curfews and how to get back at night from an evening out. Laughing, she said:

> "With my daughter, she wants all the extras, an earring here . . . in her belly button, and tattoos . . . we grit our teeth when we fight with her . . . yesterday she got a nose ring after two years of arguing with us. Boaz agreed. I didn't as much, but . . . in the end I allowed it . . . she's about to start secondary school, it'll be interesting how she'll be accepted there, if she'll succeed? . . . And the time she wants to come home is really unreasonable . . . she says, '*Everyone else* is allowed' . . . Admittedly, she says that friends accompany her, but she's not willing for us to wait for her downstairs. I'm with the phone in hand next to my ear, I say be back by 2, so at 2 the phone buzzes to wake me; if not, I call to make sure she's on her way home . . . if I don't wake, I tell her to come into our room and wake me, so I know she's back. These are all my fears relative to her."

Both parents laughed with pleasure when they described their daughter's wishes. They clearly have no difficulty uniting around anxiety that can be contained, such as their daughter returning late at night, setting boundaries, giving in after negotiation, and backing each other up. This expression of anxiety acknowledges the daughter's sexual development and that ways can be found of protecting her. However, none of the mothers mentioned these developmental issues in conflicts with sons or in relation to their sexual development, even in the form of apprehension about not getting anyone pregnant, not getting mixed up with friends who have a negative influence, not using drugs, not being violent, and so on.

The mothers' level of involvement in their daughters' lives is noticeably less than in the lives of their sons, partly because the daughters do not let them interfere.

The ideal woman

Compared to the need not to allow boys full manifestation of their abilities and to attribute fragility and vulnerability to them, girls are allowed the opportunity to express themselves freely and realize their strengths through conflict with parents. As Sara says:

> "I, myself, was surprised. A year ago the child finished with honours and a social excellence certificate. So I asked, 'What's the certificate for?', and she says, 'Whenever there's an argument, I get in the middle . . . ' She has this really developed ability to express herself, and I'm left with nothing to answer her—but it'll help her get ahead, wherever she is."

Yasmin invests a great deal of effort to ensure her boys comply with their obligations, but her sixteen-year-old daughter is responsible for her own life and serves as a successful model for the boys:

> "When Ayelet has a test, or project, she gets ready on time, she never gets pressured at the last minute. When she takes something on, a responsibility like practising her music, then she . . . plays. She wakes her brothers up, she's Miss Responsibility. Maturity as far as boys, clothes, and resistance she's only getting to now . . ."

Yasmin is able to set boundaries for her daughter while allowing her autonomy and acknowledging her sexual development.

Dina, whose oldest son is about to be recruited and whose daughter is younger, drew an idealistic image of her daughter compared to her complaints relative to her son. She described how, despite the son almost being in the army, her daughter takes on the role of "the oldest".

> "Her responsibility is greater, she's more initiating, makes decisions, and takes things on herself. From ten years old she was already babysitting . . . she can keep the house running on her own. I look at my youngest son at ten, I can't imagine . . ."

It could be that as the mothers felt, even at an unconscious level, unable to undergo a gradual releasing experience with their sons that would allow them to enjoy the boys' masculine development, they need this compensatory experience with their daughters, so they painted their daughters in idealistic hues. However, the opposite might also be true: in glorifying the daughters, the mothers do not allow them to distance themselves and grow closer to their fathers, in effect both leaving the father out of the tight family circle and raising omnipotent daughters/ women whom they can continue to control. I explore the impact of these processes on sons and daughters further on; for now it is enough to understand that if daughters are defined as ideal, it is very difficult to allow them to be themselves; in this way the dynamic of relationships between the mothers and sons also limits the space in which the daughters exist.

Notes

1. Golani Brigade, a renowned infantry brigade.
2. Special forces unit.
3. Note that when discussing universal psychic processes, the point of relevance is Western society. In other cultures, different psychic processes may occur with diverse characteristics. However, in the context of erotic feelings surfacing during breastfeeding, which is subject to physiological influence, I feel that this psychic process may cut across, and be true for all, cultures. However, this is a personal view and has no theoretical basis.
4. Rambam—acronym for Rabbi Moses ben Maimon ("Maimonides"), preeminent Jewish Bible scholar, physician, and astronomer.
5. Rambam: *Sefer Hamitzvot* (The Book of Commandments). Commandment, "You shall not".
6. *Imma*: Hebrew for mother, mum.
7. Hebrew acronym for canteen service, containing a linguistic joke by playing on the similar Hebrew word for 'rehab'—a vehicular canteen serving field soldiers.
8. *Shivah*: Hebrew for the number 7. A reference to the week spent ("sitting") at home mourning the dead.
9. Sarit and her husband's interview was not used for the study due to a technical glitch that caused it not to be recorded. They have four children, the oldest of whom was about to be recruited.
10. Based on the definition of a doctoral student from the Hebrew University who heard a lecture on the topic.
11. An onomatopoeic word describing a back and forth waving movement: equivalent to flip-flop—or, having no backbone, i.e.: wimps.
12. It was found, for example, that media violence has an inhibiting influence on violent behaviour in adolescents (Slater, Henry, Swaim, & Anderson, 2003).
13. Hebrew: father, dad.
14. Mobile canteen services.
15. Israel has a one-day weekend, Saturday, known more commonly in Israel as Sabbath.
16. Her meaning being that he should do some kind of non-commando job between 8 am and 5 pm and then return home.
17. The maternal attitude towards daughters compared to attitudes towards sons is offered to expand on the narrative told by the mothers and provide another angle.
18. Chodorow explains that in males of the oedipal stage, the decision between foregoing his own penis or foregoing his love of the parent who constitutes an object for him is sharp. He chooses his own penis, and he prefers his mother to his father, but later chooses repression in order to avoid castration. In girls things are more complex. Usually a girl does not forego her mother's love, whether as an internal or an external object, which is why daughters experience themselves as less separate than do boys and as having more porous egos. Daughters grow up and define themselves more in terms of their relationships with the other. The internalized structure of object relations becomes more complex, with more longer-term issues. These personality traits are reflected in the superego's development. Although

Freud (1905) stressed that the developmental transition leading to the choice of a sexual object is not simple, he also stressed that the description of the Oedipus complex is a schematic simplification of something deeper and more complex. It is dialectic and is also dependent on libidinal forces and accompanying psychic processes. Occasionally the daughter will, instead of identifying with the mother, defiantly choose to adopt the father's masculinity; hostility then develops towards the father rather than the mother, with a female and sexual attitude towards the mother. This situation will become increasingly complex. Additionally, the superego's growth, in both the son and the daughter, is in fact an invention of power by the psychic system in order to suppress the fierce emotions around the oedipal conflict. In both sexes, assimilation occurs (sourced in identification) with what Lacan (1956) termed "the function of the symbolic father" (who establishes the same obstacle within himself, assimilating the forbidden, boundaries, etc.).

19. Hebrew acronym for "pre-army course", which young women can choose prior to military service. These courses train for specific military roles.

CHAPTER THREE

The father's conflict

> Take now your son, your only one, whom you love, Isaac, and go you to the land of Moriah and raise him up there as an offering, on one of the mountains concerning which I will tell you . . .
>
> And he said, cast not your hand upon the lad, and do nothing to him . . .
>
> And he said, In myself I have sworn, the speech of the Lord, because you have responded with this thing, and did not withhold your son, your only one . . . I shall surely bless you, and I shall surely multiply your seed as the stars of the heavens, and as the sand upon the shore . . .
>
> Genesis 22: 1–9

In Genesis, God instructs Abraham to bind his son. When Abraham places his son on the altar and is about to kill him, an angel calls from heaven and commands him not to injure his son. Abraham's very willingness to take this action of binding merits him the blessing of generations of progeny and a nation of which he will be the starting point.

Numerous interpretations have been offered for the act of binding, from the father's preparedness to offer his son as a sacrifice for the sake of his beliefs, in testimony to the existence of murderous aggression by fathers towards their sons and the derivative feelings of guilt, through to understanding the act of binding as a warning that in order for sons to consolidate their masculine separate identities and become fathers themselves, both need to cope with the murderous, aggressive urges of father towards son. The father must be able to contain and control these instincts and be willing to acknowledge the son's total separateness.

A parallel narrative is that of Laius' attempt to kill Oedipus whose continuation constitutes the basis for understanding the development of a separate masculine identity, according to Freud. In the interviews of the fathers in this study, these motifs, appearing consciously or unconsciously, take on a particularly unique and complicated meaning in the Israeli reality.

Very few studies have focused on the psychic processes involved in military service (Ben-Ari, 2001; Lomsky-Feder & Ben-Ari, 1999; Sasson-Levy, 2006), and none have attempted to evaluate the emotional processes that fathers raising sons cope with, knowing that the sons will enter into military service and all it involves. This is the subject of this chapter.

The fathers, aged between thirty and fifty-five, had grown up in Israel and served in the army during periods of war or military activity. The knowledge that their sons will also serve accompanies them, both as fathers of sons and as spousal partners; a range of emotions, often conflicting, derive from their personal experience.

In the interviews, two patterns recur: the fathers barely spoke, and they were almost completely silent when the main topic moved to their sons' future recruitment. As explained in chapter two, one of the data analysis stages was conducted by listening to the interviewees' "first-person voice" through the "I-Poem" (Gilligan, 2002). Observing the "I-Poem" comparison tables,[1] I was surprised to discover that although when they discussed general topics around raising their children there were several "I" sentences by both parents, once the couple began talking about their son's future recruitment it was only the mothers' columns that were filled up; the fathers' columns held no, or only a very few, sentences. In Ella and Eitan's interview, for example, most of the "I-Poem" is Ella's and revolves around fears of loss of her sons, compared to only 6 (35%) of Eitan's 17 (100%) sentences. In Odelia and Oren's interview, 29 of the 46 sentences relate directly to their sons' future recruitment. Odelia speaks in all (100%) of them, whereas Oren speaks in only 14 (30%) but relates to general topics connected with raising children.

Similarly, in the 26 listings in the interview with Leah and Lapid, Leah related to anxiety relative to her older son, who was about to enlist. In contrast, Lapid expressed anxiety relative to his children in general, and his son facing recruitment, in just 8 listings. Of these, he openly expressed himself in just 4. Lapid's anxiety manifested through the feeling that it was not legitimate to voice his anxiety. The "I" sentence opening this topic, and repeated in several variations, was: "I shouldn't say what I'm about to say."

The fathers' silence can be understood from several perspectives. In Western society in general, fathers tend to be more silent (Layland, 1985). In contrast, it can be claimed that changes are occurring that culturally permit expression of emotion even by masculine men (Morman & Floyd, 2002; Peterson & Steinmetz, 2000); this could be countered, however, by claiming that Israeli society still upholds the Western world's old norms. But this does not take into consideration that Israeli paternal behaviours, as encountered by the sons overtly or covertly, may be different from those of peers in Western society, since they derive from unconscious emotional dynamics unique to Israeli society. The fact that similar behaviour is the convention elsewhere in the world may serve as a defence mechanism against deep acknowledgment of the unique messages in Israeli society and the consequences to which they give rise.

The paternal silence is evidence of an emotional pattern that Ben-Ari (1998) termed "masking-up". He relates it to the problematic policing roles of army reservists in the midst of Palestinian populations: donning a mask allows the reservists to separate themselves from reality. He describes how the reservists become "others" as they create a distinction between their functioning in the temporary military environment and in the permanent public-civilian environment, as a way of balancing the contrast between the two and suspending their civilian orientation. They can thus provide themselves with the authorization for behaviour different from their civilian patterns. The dissonance in military functioning is not only the problem but, to a certain extent, also the solution: it allows the reservist to function from a painful awareness of the practical outcomes and to separate civilian from military consciousness. This dissociation, in psychoanalytic terms, makes it harder for them to bring this aspect of themselves into their fatherhood and explains an additional aspect of paternal silence.

In research focused on the perception of fatherhood among adolescent males in Israel, Pelach-Galil (2004) found that fathers are absent from their sons' emotional lives, leaving the sons with an emotional deficiency and sense of distress. There was a sense of guilt—often not conscious—towards their sons who must enlist; as Yair Lapid, former journalist and finance minister, wrote on the eve of his son's recruitment: "I'm familiar with so many moments of the coming years, and there's nothing I can do. . . . I can't protect you this time, my child."[2]

But the discourse above does not shed light on the multilevel and multidimensional unconscious and conscious emotional platform causing fatherhood silence, or on the consequences of this on sons and their masculine identity—topics we explore in this chapter.

Manifestations of fatherhood loss anxiety

In a letter sent to his son prior to the latter's recruitment, Yair Lapid expressed his anxiety over his son's recruitment through the voice of his son's mother: "Your mother phoned yesterday crying and said that you'd received your first call-up papers." This image recurred in the interviews with the parents. Most of the fathers did not openly express their anxiety towards their sons relative to future recruitment but did expand on the fact that "the mothers" are anxious. As we saw, the mothers cooperated and voiced the anxiety. Some sons absorbed this and expressed anxiety about the time when they would be grown and serving in the military.

Boaz was different. He said that anxiety accompanied him from the moment of his son's birth, and that he opposes his son serving as a combatant. It is interesting to note, however, that without realizing it, he spoke in the feminine form (Hebrew contains male and female forms for all words but adverbs), perhaps to distance the anxiety:

> "It's something that you've thought about all these years. Each time you have a child, you say, 'By the time he gets to the army it'll probably be calm' . . . you always say, all the time there's talk about the army. It surrounds you, at home or with friends . . . You always think about how it will be when he's recruited . . . even when he went to study computers you thought about when he goes to the army, and he won't go to a commando unit, he'll be in computers. That's how it is . . ."

Other fathers tried to neutralize anxiety by using derogation or through contradictory sentences—like Eitan, father of three young sons, who was silent for most of the interview:

> "I don't agree with what she thinks about the army . . . I think it's possible to . . . gain from the three years, those who go for the officer's course profit from taking that direction . . ."

and then immediately contradicted himself:

> "There's no doubt . . . that there's risk, it's a system with some not so nice or pleasant aspects, and there are also some dangerous

things . . . But going to the jungle is no less dangerous than being in the army."

Lapid would talk about the feelings flooding him on Memorial Day only when his wife Leah left the room. Even so, he did not talk openly about his son; he spoke about one of the neighbourhood boys who fell in battle, emphasizing twice that Leah does not know about his feelings. This information was accompanied by agitated movements, compared with the greater body control accompanying his other remarks or that of other fathers in control of their emotions. This pattern is consistent with the familiar masculine image in Western society, which is similar to the ideal combat masculinity and in Israel is further impacted by military codes of control and overcoming emotion (Sasson-Levy, 2006).

Lapid also found it easier to express his fear through his wife. When, through projective identification, the fear is handed over to her, he can resist it, on the one hand, and calm it, on the other. He explained:

> "I . . . am not as sensitive as she is. I am sensitive, but not like her. I have a problem on memorial days, it's my crowd, with all the stories . . . but I leave it here inside . . ."

And he pointed to the left side of his chest. Oren expressed a similar stance:

> "Most of my friends still don't have sons in the army . . . I think gender sets how men and women cope with this kind of thing . . . Men don't talk about it, they push it under the carpet or something, and they get ulcers or heart attacks."

The gesture with which Lapid ended his words, touching his hand to his heart as though it encloses his pain, and the statement with which Oren closed his remarks, are chilling. Yet despite Oren's awareness of the price men pay for not expressing emotion, he could not behave differently "from his kind" and found an outlet for his fear by displacing it (A. Freud, 1936) and expressing it through the sons:

> "I think Ori said he's afraid, . . . his solution is to want to be a medic in the medical corps . . . when any of us goes anywhere, he gets really scared."

The muteness of the fathers

Looking only at the revealed content in the fathers' words, we might conclude that they did not share what they experienced during military service, or that their service was not significant. But since they served in the military in both the compulsory service and as reservists through several wars, their experience is a central component in shaping their personalities. Knowing that Israeli men tend to recall their military service fondly, keep social connections formed during service, and relate army tales, especially when in each other's company (Ben-Ari, 2001; Lieblich, 1989; Lomsky-Feder, 1992; Sasson-Levy, 2006), their silence on this issue, particularly as their own sons are about to undergo similar experiences, is questionable.

The few sentences spoken by the fathers were said in a cold, matter-of-fact tone. Sefi, father of three sons and two daughters, just gave the name of the unit he served in and said that when there's no choice, one must simply function; there's no room for emotions.

Complex emotional dynamics are the background to the fathers' silence relative to military recruitment in their life stories. I needed to listen to the meaning of this silence, and the nuances surfacing from within it, in order to discern whether their memories and narratives contained traumatic experiences or experiences of satisfaction and achievement, and how the way they were engraved in their internal worlds related to their fathering of sons. What message do the fathers convey through their silence?

Had I not already known the extent of emotional storm in statements such as, *I served in the Lebanon War . . . I was a commando with all that that involves . . . I was injured by shrapnel . . .*, I could easily have thought, erroneously, that we were talking about peripheral events of little importance, as when Hillel muttered, in reaction to Hedy's anxiety: "No . . . I was in Lebanon but . . . I was there exactly when the war started . . ."

I felt how difficult it was for him, so I asked, "In which corps?" He continued talking quietly, eyes looking down: "Paratroopers . . . commando and all that . . . less frightening . . . but it is frightening, yeah."

Rafael only spoke after Ruth said: "His mother told me that the three of them were in the army at the same time. Three soldiers! Can you imagine that?! She said it was the hardest time of her life, she just didn't sleep!"

Then Rafael added: "I don't know how it's possible to cope . . . not just regular army . . . but war."

In this way I could see that Rafael had served in the military during a very difficult war period. We can assume the consequences and influences this experience had on his outlook on life and death, but the details of what he did and experienced during his military service remained hidden from view.

Unlike the mothers, who wanted to distance their sons from military service, the fathers expressed conflict. Zak said:

> "I grew up in a period when . . . nationalism was strong . . . after the Six Day War . . . My two brothers and I were officers together in the army, it gave our parents and us a feeling of prestige and pride . . . I had really high motivation to serve in the army, I wanted to go into all kinds of high-level things. I started out in combat units, in tanks, but some months later, because of a medical problem, I became a jobnik . . . My kids will be influenced by that same phenomenon . . . of going for elite units, that's actually what will happen to my kids."

From Zak's remarks, it becomes apparent that the essence of his masculine identity and shaping of his personality that also await his sons and mean danger to their lives influences his reaction as a father:

> "If they do actually go to super-commando, then I'll assure them through personal example from my jobnik period."

Weighed against the anxiety that his combat period would serve as a personal example to his sons, who may adopt his values and endanger their lives, comes Zak's self-calming statement that his "jobnik" days can also serve as another personal example to his sons and one that preserves life.

Boaz, whose son was shortly to be recruited, felt he was expressing a feeling shared by fathers of sons:

> "Every father thinks . . . that if we could do the army instead of our kids, we would . . ."

Boaz went into more detail:

> "I was in reconnaissance. We went through things I don't want my son to go through. I wouldn't want him going through the Casbah,[3] it's so dangerous . . . I wouldn't want to risk even a fingernail of his. And, ideologically, I don't really believe in it so much now."

Then his conflict surfaced:

> "It's not fair to say I don't want to send my son. On the other hand, I know exactly what the army is, I'm familiar with the dangers. And when I told him this, he said, 'After your military service, you have no right to say that to me.' I didn't answer him . . . what can I say?"

Becca echoes: "There's nothing to say."

Boaz continued:

> "He says to me, you were in that particular unit, and you come to me expecting me to be a jobnik?"

Boaz shared the distress apparent in the other fathers' comments: that because he served in an elite unit, he has lost—in his own, his wife's, and his son's view—the fatherly right to direct his son in a way that protects his life.

Dina never stopped expressing her anxiety about her son's upcoming recruitment, but her husband, David, was mostly silent. Initially he said only a few words, but his openness gradually increased on encountering emotions previously unexpressed openly and consciously:

> "I think that serving in the army is the right thing to do. I felt shit when some of my friends' sons started expressing doubt about whether they should serve at all, and especially not in elite units . . . I found that so upsetting . . . here in our country we can't allow ourselves . . ."

What appear to be values, however, perhaps reveal themselves to be feelings of guilt. His words present a paradoxical conflict embedded in the very definition of the role of the father (which I expand on later): David adopted the values of military service in order to protect his homeland, which includes his family; however, his protective actions clearly contain risk, which he realizes might present itself as his son making decisions to please the father:

> "If he does it only to please me, then . . . maybe I'll feel guilt. I want it to come from him. He should know it's something that *he* must do . . . otherwise it really will be tough for me."

David continued, quietly:

> "They asked me, 'Abba, did you shoot? . . . And kill, and all that?' so I always tried to evade that . . . I don't feel like . . . that I like to think about that I did, even to myself, and of course I'm not comfortable talking to them about it . . . to no one, and of course not to the kids."

It seems that David was not able to integrate his military experience as a soldier who killed into his everyday persona. Therefore, since he wishes this part of him had never existed, his silence also functions towards himself. Almost another hour of interview passed until an additional reason for the silence was revealed:

> "These are also . . . tough situations, where you almost break, it's so, so hard. So I don't . . . maybe I was a little scared . . . to tell them, maybe I was scared . . . that . . . they'll be afraid of it . . ."

Then he detailed:

> "Everyone talks about heroes. No one talks about it, but in every war there are plenty who don't function, they don't get up at all . . . I don't know if it's even possible to prepare someone for that."

David tries to calm himself:

> "I hope it won't be bad for them, I'm not made of anything different to what they are. Yariv will go through it better than I did . . . people are revealed in situations like that, they discover strengths that come, they have no clue from where . . ."

Yet experiences of death, fear, and helplessness flooded him:

> "Look, the fear.. if you haven't experienced fear . . . fear of dying, I don't know . . . when you're facing it, and you know that a percentage of the people . . . won't go back . . . it's a frightening idea not to come back or to get severely injured or become disabled, so it's hard to . . . talk about. Anyhow, what's that good for . . . that they'll get frightened because of it? They're growing up and they'll need to deal with it . . . I don't know if it's possible to prepare themselves for things . . . I hope they won't need to go through it, but if they do . . . I don't know if it helps to prepare someone? When you get to it, either you function, or not."

Therefore, David's solution is silence, and silencing: "When it comes up, I try to distance . . . I try not to think about it."

Oren said, of himself, that he has strong awareness and verbal abilities. Relative to other fathers, he spoke in depth, making it possible to understand what others had expressed in similar terms but with far less clarity. His pauses conveyed to me that these were things he found difficult to talk about:

> "There is tension between two ways of looking at my military experiences . . . I have very positive experiences, relative to what I did . . . gratification, contributing, and so on. Additionally, there's the ideological aspect, being committed to the need to serve, and so on . . . But because of the danger, there's also a fear relative to myself in the past and my children in the future. There's a conflict between us around each of the children . . . on stances to do with the army. Odelia manifests one side of the coin and I the other, but

> we hold the same coin . . . I'm sure when one of my sons goes to the army, it'll be traumatic for me too . . . perhaps as much as . . . or more difficult than for Odelia, even though we may express it in different ways."

I asked: "Does this influence your fathering in any way?" From Oren's response it was evident that the feelings and thoughts were difficult for him:

> "I think . . . that with my sons . . . I try a little less to express my positive army experiences and my feelings about the importance of military service . . . I think that's because . . . the difficulty of the situation we're in, between Odelia and myself, and each of us within ourselves."

In other words, Oren explained that he does not share this important experience in his life and his ideological views with his sons because of anxiety over his sons' lives and his conflict with his wife.

Sefi was mostly silent; when he did speak, he noted the division of roles between mothers and fathers, something I had found among the couples. He expresses his anxiety through the mother, who keeps the son close by, compared to himself, who is committed to military service.

> "No mother of any soldier . . . can watch her sons going through difficult experiences . . . but that's part of the army activities, nothing can be done . . . somebody's got to do it. So that we can live in this country. Israel means army. They're linked. It's part of our framework. Everything you do in your life touches on this issue of the army in some way. So . . . if you aren't connected with the army, or weren't in the army, you have no place in our society."

I had thought that the idea of life following release from the army contains a message of optimism and would contain the anxiety for his life. Nonetheless, I understood him saying "There's no such thing as a mother who'd send her sons to the army with a calm heart" as a projection of his anxiety, so I asked: "Is that something that goes through your mind?" He answered:

> "Sure . . . every so often it passes through my thoughts when you see certain kinds of events on TV or read about them in the papers, something that happened to soldiers, then you say, I'll be at that stage in another three, four years."

Yitzhak's contradictions and truncated sentences were a different kind of anxiety silencing and expressed unresolved conflict.

"No . . . yes, enlisting seems obvious to me . . . but it's not logical that you endanger the boys . . . even though in my view military service is an experience . . . and it gives you so much . . . but, everyone wants their son not to experience . . . dangers . . . they have a good example from home, we don't persuade them not to go into the army, on the contrary, I did reserve duty up to the last moment."

Yitzhak and Yasmin described behaviours in their boys that they find unacceptable—insolence to teachers, not preparing homework, and so on. But I also caught an opposite message, one of satisfaction that their sons do not accept the system's rules. They had sent their children to a school that was known for having pupils who are also non-conformist relative to military duty. I began to wonder: could it be that, unconsciously, they are encouraging non-conformist behaviour in their son, as a way of paving the way to his decision not to serve? If this is correct, in what kind of complicated position is the son put when he cannot understand which message he should obey in order to please his parents while consolidating his own values? Is the message "it's necessary to live with dual messages"? Perhaps this is the way Yitzhak found to cope with the conflict between his fear and wish to protect his sons, and his values.

The silence of fathers wounded during military service

Both David and Lapid were wounded during their military service. Their attitudes towards their injuries differ, but the emotional message conveyed was identical. Lapid talked about his injury in detail, showing a large scar on his arm. David did not mention anything: Dina was the one who, carefully choosing her words, brought up the subject. In their different ways, both men conveyed a similar emotional message that celebrates the virtue of overcoming the difficulty. They didn't talk about pain, or the complexity of a young man coping with more than light injury. Their words did not contain expressions of weakness, or any emotional expression at all. There is silence also in this context. For example, all Dina said was: "David was, um, . . . wounded in the army."

There was something about the way she said this that suggested I should continue the conversation, so I asked: "What happened? How were you injured?"

David: "I wasn't injured badly, but I was wounded in the Yom Kippur War . . ."

Dina: "And in the . . ."

David: "I was injured in the Gulf War."

Dina: "Yes . . ."

"What happened to you?" I asked.

David: "In the Yom Kippur War I got hit by shrapnel, here . . ."

David showed me the scars on his left arm. He spoke in a nonchalant tone, as though implying "it's nothing, no need to make a fuss".

"I was flat on my back for some three weeks . . ."

Reacting to his tone, I responded with humour: "A very simple thing." We all laughed, perhaps to reduce the tension. Then Dina spoke, tapping her right hand lightly on her right cheek:

"Yes . . . very simple . . . and afterwards in Gaza."

I repeated: "Very simple . . ." They laughed again, and David seemed pleased that his facial injury was being taken more seriously than the way he felt he should present it. He pointed to all the changes on the side of his face, explaining:

"All of this area was reconstructed . . ."

The look on my face must have disclosed the pain I felt on realizing he was actually quite severely wounded, and David closed that conversation, as though comforting me, by saying:

"But it looks better now than it did before."

Dina took control over her agitated emotions and continued talking about her fears for her firstborn, about to enlist, and her boys in general, who may take David as an example and join commando units. Perhaps David's emotional code, which ignores the difficult emotional and physical coping he experienced, made it easier for Dina to continue casting responsibility for their sons' lives on him. Perhaps for his part and facing that reality, silencing emotions is the only way possible.

Lapid, whose son was also on the verge of recruitment, was injured during his military service at the level known as "medium", but it changed the course of his life. He had to alter his career path, met and married his wife, and began life as father and head of the household. Following his injury, he found himself needing the assistance of others. His laconic way of describing the event is similar to David's:

> "I did the army, like everyone else. I was in tanks. I was injured during reserve duty in '82 . . . right at the start of the war."

Leah was clearly filled with pain. Interestingly, my own reaction was similar: even though Lapid's words aroused strong emotions in me, I forced myself to contain and enclose them, perhaps using, in some unconscious way, the unspoken code pervading the room.

> "And . . . during my hospitalization . . . I met Leah."

With his right hand, he touched Leah's arm. Taking into account the significant impact of the injury on his life, it is evident that he has adopted coping patterns that do not allow for emotion at all, particularly not self-pity. Lapid only expanded on the subject in response to my direct question, and his words are focused on being nothing more than informative:

> "My whole left side was injured, my left leg . . ."

I asked him how it happened.

> "An attack by jets . . . my left hand was a total mess, now it's okay, more or less."

He opened and closed his left hand, showing that it's fine, and then immediately shifted to the positive aspects of the injury:

> "So I was wounded . . . but I met her . . ."

Later Lapid returned to the circumstances of his injury, and his remarks caused a sense of extreme helplessness:

> "Being helpless is the toughest thing, I suffer from it, because my injury was from a state of being helpless. If I'd been injured by Syrian forces, shooting at me . . . then at least . . . But here, I couldn't do a thing against it, it was our own forces . . ."

Lapid closed his hands into fists.

> "I didn't go into rehab and all that stuff. The kids came, work, income. I changed my profession, I left computers because of my wounds . . . so I went to study, I did okay in that area too . . . I didn't have any complaints. In short, I found myself."

Clearly, in the Israeli reality the silence of the fathers carries unique significance connected with emotional processes undergone when facing their sons' recruitment. Some silenced emotions and disturbing memories from their military service days that they found difficult to integrate into their personalities; some were silent based on a feeling that there was no way to prepare their sons for what they would encounter; some were silenced by a feeling of guilt that their actions and personal example might bring their sons closer to death; some were silenced for this reason by their wives, some were silenced by their sons.

Even the wounded fathers who underwent exhausting rehabilitation procedures were silent over the events that had caused their injuries and silenced the emotions that did not correspond with independent abilities to overcome the difficulties. The characteristics of silence hone the understanding that this could be a characteristic of Israeli fathering of sons, deriving from the emotional stress with which Israeli fathers must cope, *a stress that has so far not been considered.*

The Binding of Isaac

One myth directly relating to Israeli fathers revolves around the narrative of the Binding of Isaac. It is central to Jewish–Israeli emotional baggage in the context of fathers sending their sons into the army. This concept is therefore to varying degrees of consciousness at the back of Israeli fathers' minds. Before discussing the meaning of the fathers' comments as those surfaced in the study, I wish to present the way in which two professors of social science, both of whom lost sons in military action, relate to the myth: Shlomo Giora Shoham (1998, 2005), and Mordechai Rotenberg (2003). Their theories shed light on and provide meaning to a concealed layer of emotional coping in Israeli fathers of sons. At an event in his honour, Professor Rotenberg said:

> We must understand . . . Abraham's knife as Damocles' sword, both stimulating and strengthening, which should ensure continuity of ideological belief and the promised progress . . . despite, or because of, the sharp blade laid across the neck.

Avshalom Elitzur (2003) explained Rotenberg's perspective:

> Rotenberg views Isaac's binding as a message that fortifies the sons and gives them the tools that allow them to continue living under conditions of threat to their physical or economic existence in situations when they are not protected by their parents but stand, themselves, exposed.

Shoham (1998, 2005) reads the narrative of the binding as the opposite, terrible commandment, "slay your son", and of course he relates to the unconscious processes:

> A burnt offering must be beautiful, healthy and perfect. The macabre analogy is that only the healthy, the best, and the whole in body and soul go to the air force, the reconnaissance units, and the other elite commando units. . . . In our context, we can view the father as identifying with his dead son, that embodiment of his young image. In his death, the son unites with eternity, and through him the father, by extended identification, also attains unity with perfection . . . the final paradox, then, is that the myth of the binding causes the sacrifice of the choicest, beautiful, excellent young men not for the sake of the deity's perfection but to the Moloch of mediocrity. [Shoham, 1998]

In my opinion, Rotenberg and Shoham have dared to look complex psychic layers in the eye, so to speak, and cope with feelings of guilt, which surfaced in this study too—feelings that accompany the fathers in the reality where the sons risk their lives during military service, where the fathers who raised the sons through personal example and value-based education fill a central role in realizing this reality.

Another father coping with similar emotions in the face of his son's recruitment is Freud himself, who described his dream:

> Indistinct beginning. *I tell my wife I have some news for her, something very special. She becomes frightened, and does not wish to hear it. I assure her that on the contrary it is something which will please her greatly, and I begin to tell her that our son's Officers' Corps has sent a sum of money (5,000 k.?) . . . something about honourable mention . . . distribution . . . at the same time I have gone with her into a sitting room, like a store-room, in order to fetch something from it. Suddenly I see my son appear; he is not in uniform but rather in a tight-fitting sports suit (like a seal?) with a small cap. He climbs on to a basket which stands to one side near a chest, in order to put something on this chest. I address him; no answer. It seems to me that his face or forehead is bandaged, he arranges something in his mouth, pushing something into it. Also his hair shows a glint of grey. I reflect: Can he be so exhausted? And has he false teeth?* Before I can address him again I awake without anxiety, but with palpitations. My clock points to 2.30 a.m. [1900, pp. 397–398; emphasis in original]

As Freud explains, he is conscious of the anxiety, which he describes as "distressing expectations", over his son fighting on the front, and he copes with the anxiety through its inverse: "At the start of the dream we see the energetic effort to exchange the sorrowful thoughts for their opposite." In seeking the source of the anxiety as an expression of an unconscious wish/conflict, he identifies the existence of the unconscious wish for his son's death as embedded in the basis of the dream. But, unlike Shoham's statement, Freud understood this terrible wish as being a means of dulling the pain that would arise should he need to cope with his son's death.

Elitzur relates to the force of resistance with which Freud needs to cope in his efforts to reach the root of the wish for his son's death that forms the basis of the dream, and the force of internal resistance with which he needed to struggle during the course of his attempts to reach this understanding. He links this understanding to his own experiences as a university lecturer: almost every time he taught this dream, listeners with sons in the military reacted to it with harsh comments, describing Freud as someone with pathological wishes, wondering how he dared to apply them to others. They would furiously protest against the claim that fathers could be wishing death on their sons. Elitzur states that this criticism is inconsistent with human culture, which is hardly innocent of paedocide in the name of one or another deity, such as that in the narrative of the Binding of Isaac.

The raw texts of Freud, Shlomo Giora Shoham, and Elitzur, which point to the potential existence of difficult-to-cope-with unconscious destructive forces in the father's psyche relative to the son, bring to mind such forces in Greek mythology.

If we observe the myth narratives as representing psychic structures and dynamics, we can understand them as representing the parenthood–couple relationship dynamic: when control over the father's ability for restraint, and its force, are lost, it endangers the future; at this stage the mother needs to intervene. Uranus and Gaia, the first couple in mythology, gave birth, among their other children, to the Titans. Uranus, the first father-figure in Greek mythology, loathed Gaia's fertility, the earth, and did not allow it to see the light of day. Gaia suffered from Uranus' violence and called on her adult sons, the Titans, for help. According to Hesiod, Uranus' violence towards his offspring is the first evil, cause of all evil thereafter, the first sin of the father deity, destined to recur throughout following generations (Shinoda-Bolen, 2002, p. 38). Of the sons, Cronus (who represents time) castrated his father, thereby halting the father's action. Cronus then became the strongest male deity.

The image of Cronus is closer to that of the human father, but he is nonetheless a terrible father. He is characterized by wanting order, regime, history, structured layering, and principles. As an ancient astrological personality theory, this type of father figure matches that of the strict father in Western culture and classic psychoanalysis. But Cronus is too powerful and must become refined. Fearing his own children will do to him what he did to his father, he swallows them.

His behaviour is different from that of Uranus, who buried his offspring in the mother's belly: Cronus brings them into his own self, with all the symbolic significance implied by this act. These narratives, says Shinoda-Bolen (2002, p. 39), are a metaphorical way for the father to prevent his offspring from rising higher than he or challenging his stances or beliefs.

With these narratives and Freud's dream in mind when we relate the oedipal narrative, which Freud turned into a symbol of the stage of masculine development in which the son wishes to kill the father in order to turn himself into a man, it is surprising that Freud ignored the stage that precedes Oedipus' wish to kill his father. This is the stage in which Laius, King of Thebes, hears from the Delphic Oracle that if he had a child, it would kill him. To prevent that event, after Oedipus' birth Laius drives a shaft into his son's ankle and orders one of the shepherds to abandon him in a desolate part of Mount Cithaeron, in order to kill him (Shabtai, 2000). Findings of studies on father–son relationships indeed describe the existence of contradictory feelings and wishes in these relationships (Esman, 1985; Hunter & Youniss, 1982; Pelach-Galil, 2004; Shulman & Seiffge-Krenke, 1997; Yogman, 1982).

These primal instinctive forces exist as unconscious raw potential in the human psyche. When Israeli fathers find themselves required to send their sons to the army, into potentially life-threatening situations, this requirement may project onto those same unconscious forces and rouse them from their slumber; by their very arousal, they then threaten the emotional equilibrium needed by the fathers to uphold their paternal role.

The intergenerational and intercultural baggage carried into the psyche of the mythological father, together with the acknowledgment of the possibility of arousing unconscious underground activity of that kind in the fatherhood psyche, echo in the meaning behind what the fathers say. From this perspective, the fathers' silence can be understood as an attempt, through avoidance, of trying to again take control of primal forces rising in them as a consequence of living in a country where sons must be sent into the army. This defence mechanism causes their muteness/disappearance as fathers precisely when their sons need them the most—during adolescence.

Thus, maternal behaviour that keeps the son close both while resisting the son's development into a warrior-man and also distancing the son from the father, protects both father and son: the son, against the father's aggressive feelings; the father, against the need to cope with agitating feelings embedded in his unconscious. Through silence, the father cooperates with this analogous pattern.

Guilt feelings

The fathers directly expressed feelings of guilt towards their sons. I encountered behaviours towards sons that can be understood as compensatory and overprotective, or waiving demands and boundaries, as in Rafael's perception that he must ensure things are always pleasant and good for his children and must change any reality that does not comply; or the approach of Yitzhak, who wanted to prevent his children from experiencing any psychic unpleasantness.

To prevent the children from not feeling good—and perhaps as an outlet for his unconscious conflictual feelings—Yitzhak talked about how he gives to his children without limits and without demands. When I asked: "To make them feel good?" he smiled and said: "Yes, that's part of the protectiveness." In Hebrew, this last word carries a dual meaning: nursery school-type behaviour, alluding to the tendency in the maternal approach to sons that attempts to halt the process of development from boy into man; and the defensive behaviour of overprotectiveness and excessive giving.

Guilt feelings worked their way into Lapid's words through transference of responsibility to government:

> I am, after all, just a citizen. In this country . . . it's helplessness. Yes. *Because if I know I did something wrong*, then maybe I can fix it, but I can't . . . I have no way of controlling it."

The labyrinth of unresolvable fatherhood conflict

The psychic stress with which the Israeli father needs to cope is weighty and complex. Further on we discuss the unconscious intergenerational emotional baggage it contains, but the current reality is not simple and locks the father into a booby-trapped emotional conflict.

Fathers have two basic functions: protecting the family from the outside world while (1) ensuring the safety of their children and (2) gradually allowing external reality into the protected mother–child relationship (Target & Fonagy, 2002). With sons, the father's role is to help them shape their separate masculine identity by, among other things, being the role and identity model.

And herein lies the conflict: to take part in protecting the family when faced with the ongoing threat to Israel's security and very existence from elements hostile to it, coupled with the history of persecution and calamity in the Jewish people, the fathers adopt a political-ideological and values perception that sides with recruitment into the army to protect the country and thereby their families. But those same perceptions, which require recruitment of their sons at age eighteen and their combat service, instantly turns the protective mechanism into an endangering one. However, if in order to protect their sons, the fathers abandon these values and adopt approaches that enable evasion of military service, they will need to cope with the question of "Who will fight, who will protect the family?" The conflict also appears in connection with the developmental role of fathers relative to sons. These fathers, who have themselves undergone the stages of shaping as men through dangerous military activities, based on the masculine-combat model, cannot present themselves to their sons as examples and role models: if they do, they again find themselves bringing their sons into danger.

Additionally, by virtue of the fathers being Israeli men, they are responsible for their sons' recruitment and thereby for endangering their sons' lives, which arouses a dormant unconscious emotional dynamic experienced as the wish for the son's death—a dynamic that, without the need to cope with the conflict, would lie undisturbed in the psyche's unconscious.

Being trapped in conflictual forces relative to their emotional basis as fathers, the Israeli fathers experience harsh emotions: the trap is so difficult that the natural way of coping is through patterns of avoidance, manifested, among others, in silence, stammering, and unclear emotional expressions.

Explicit expressions of helplessness and loss anxiety in the fathers' conversations

Some of the fathers allow themselves to express helplessness, primarily in light of the fact that they cannot serve in place of their sons, knowing that there is no sure way to ready the sons for the harsh coping that may await them as soldiers, and relative to the emotional conflict in which they exist. In reaction, they have developed various outlooks.

This is demonstrated in Yair Lapid's statement earlier in this chapter: "I'm familiar with so many moments of the coming years, and there's nothing I can do."

Ruth and Rafael, for example, developed an outlook that one of their sons might die while in service. Perhaps as with Freud's dream, by trying to prepare in advance, they are attempting to feel less helpless.

Rafael's outlook may be linked to his experiences as a young soldier: we know nothing about his actual service other than that he served during an active war period. While shaking his head in negation constantly, he said:

> "Some people live to be eighty or ninety and did nothing . . . just ate, worked, never enjoyed a book, never played. Their whole life was just . . . bad. And to some people, at twenty, or even younger, things happen that . . . and everyone's so sorry, but in the end, they had a full life, with friends and experiences and . . . that's how I see the purpose of raising kids, reaching the point that at any given moment I . . . you can be satisfied with what you did so far . . ."

Sefi, who described the difficult feeling of helplessness manifesting in all areas of life, reached a similar conclusion, but instead of providing him with relief in any way, it caused him emotional stress and anxiety:

> "It's not much good making long-term plans. You need to live for the day and do . . . that is, if you've got through everything okay, then carry on with the next day. That's how I see it. Really, there's no quiet in this country, life's terrible . . . especially these days. These days, the past few weeks, it's a war of survival from all angles. So I . . . to think macro, it looks pretty bad. That's how I move forward in the meantime, let's see how long I can . . . that's it, that's it."

Yitzhak also said:

> "My whole attitude is fatalistic: 'what will be, will be'. Actually, if someone does or doesn't go into the army, it doesn't mean he'll be harmed more or harmed less. That is . . . some don't go into the army and then get killed in a traffic accident, or they serve in the command centres and then get run over . . . the likelihood of that is higher. It's all a matter of probability."

We met Lapid when he spoke about being injured by friendly fire, and how he can't bear the feeling of being helpless, unable to accept helplessness as part of reality. To resolve that, he was willing to bluntly face anxiety to restore his sense of having done something against a situation where he could lose one of his sons. But even for Lapid, it's not simple: he notes that it was his brother who had the harshest words to say:

> "Look, it should never be said, my brother . . . he said it. In our country, you must never raise just one son . . . you need more . . .

> because there's a chance you could be left with nothing . . . that's what he said. And that's with me all the time."

Leah sat, frozen, then nodded: small affirmative movements. Lapid added:

> "She said, 'How can you talk like that?' So I said to her, 'That's the reality. After all, you read the papers . . .'"

Additional emotional defences used by the fathers

We need to keep in mind that parents raised the issue of their sons' future recruitment without being specifically asked about it: so we can understand their subsequent statements as additional defence mechanisms, such as repressing the harsh emotional baggage for a future timeframe, as Eitan said:

> "That's not a topic that bothers me right now. Getting pressured about what will be in another ten years looks to me a bit unrealistic. Maybe by then . . . there'll be peace. And maybe the opposite. I'm not thinking forward to then right now."

Zak's line of thought is similar:

> "Thinking about twenty years ahead is a bit too far for us. Right now, we're in nappies, it's peepee and poopoo. We're relatively older . . . maybe there'll be another child, so at fifty I'll still be dealing with pee and poo . . . the timeframe of army is a long way off at this point."

Sefi noted a chilling reason for focusing on the present: the fear that there won't be a future.

> "I believe in a fatalistic approach: that what will happen, will. You can't fight it. . . . That's how I deal with things. One day at a time, without too much looking ahead and thoughts about what will be or not be . . . *because maybe it'll be won't be.* In my view, that's the best way of coping . . . taking a deep breath."

Hillel also said he only thought short-term, not about the army at all. But his fears did not disappear, and he tried to distance them with talk of generalities. That didn't help either; an additional defence appeared in the form of rationalization: logical reasons for why boys should not serve in combat units. The transparency of this defence is greater, because even as a smart, rational person, Hillel is not successful at following a simple, logical line of thought on this issue. "If I try to analyse it for myself, then I wouldn't want that, because it's not healthy to be there . . ."

This reason was traded for a different, "logical" reason:

> "*Of course I don't decide for them.* If asked, I'll say that from my experience it's better not to go for combat units—not because it's dangerous . . . but simply *because it's less interesting.* Being a combatant means *three years drying out your brain.* Today there are brigades where you can contribute as much: computers, intelligence . . . If there's no choice, someone's . . . *but if they ask me, I'll tell them to let someone else do it."*

Hillel was noticeably protecting himself from being conscious of the impossible situation he is in as a father who, based on his values and his understanding of the Israeli reality and on his experiences, needs to guide his sons to recruitment roles that could endanger their lives.

My dad's a hero

According to Lapid, the reason for his emotional restraint and concealing of fears is connected with his role as a father.

> "When you see some moving documentary on Memorial Day, then if a tear comes . . . I don't let the kids see tears in my eyes, ever."

I asked: "Why not?"

> "Because it's not good! There's nothing greater for a boy than his dad, so should he see his father crying? . . . it'll hamper his self-confidence."

Lapid spoke about his little boy's anxieties. I wondered whether Lapid might have passed his unprocessed fears on to his son—perhaps Lapid feels guilty about that. Lapid continued, and I understood more:

> "On several occasion he asked me . . . the little one, 'Abba, what would you do?' He knows I have a gun which is either in the safe or under the pillow, depending on what I sense . . . So he asks, 'Why's the gun under the pillow?' or his next question was, 'Abba, what will you do if an Arab comes and . . .?' I said to him, 'Nothing. The Arab won't do anything. Not all of them are bad.' He says, 'No, Abba, if he comes to shoot us.' So I said, 'If he comes to shoot us, I've got a gun. I'll do what needs . . .' 'Will you shoot at him?' 'Yes, I suppose . . . I'll have to hit him. Of course I'll try to get him.' For a kid of six to think of things like this is not good, it's really terrible.

You ask yourself again: What? What kind of world are we bringing our kids into?"

This interview took place in July 2002, during a period of multiple terror attacks, often in places milling with people. Some terrorists entered homes and murdered everyone. As a result, many Israeli men equipped themselves with guns. Nonetheless, Lapid's behaviour, in sometimes placing the gun under his pillow, is somewhat irregular for a person living in the central region of Israel. One wonders whether he is suffering from undiagnosed post-trauma stress, because his behaviour is otherwise functional.

It seems that Lapid unconsciously senses he suffers from anxiety and is passing it on to his young son. He tried to balance this with the message that "not all Arabs are bad", but the boy clarified his intention precisely, seemingly verbalizing his father's fears: he meant an Arab who had come to kill them. To Lapid's response "I've got a gun. I'll do what needs . . .", the son interrupts and asks for clarification: "Will you shoot him?" Lapid's difficulty in answering this question conveys to the child, albeit unconsciously, how difficult this subject is for his father.

Throughout the interview, Lapid repeated and emphasized that he is strong, and that he must appear strong to his family. The statements in which Lapid expresses his fears clarifies that he is in deep emotional stress. The disparity between his fears and the strong façade he presents to his family only adds to the difficulty. Being flooded with so much anxiety around his children gave me the feeling that Lapid is unable to contain his anxiety, which spills into almost every sphere of his life. The following remarks came from the whole interview, with linking words added to make them into a coherent whole:

"Every age has its fears. Fear of the streets . . . drugs. We were afraid the little one was hyperactive, but that turned out to be rubbish. The fear of failing. An unsuccessful child is your failure. The whole situation's a bit frightening . . . it never should be said . . . but today I'd think twice about bringing kids into the world. I'm talking now about here, in Israel. You fear for your kids' lives . . . let's say it openly: what's his chance of coming back from the army, or getting injured? So now the boundary is blurred . . . between front-lines and home front. Because in retrospect, I think more civilians were wounded than soldiers. It's frightening to raise kids here, it's really worrying . . . There's also the fear that the country won't exist, that there's no hope, since it became a country with no values, with an ultra-Orthodox population that doesn't bear its share of the economic and security burden, with a problematic demographic

> compared with the Arab culture. It's really frightening. Very worrying ... it's hard to see the light. So there's this breaking point, in me too ... that here we will always be at war. But there's no choice ... that's what there is ... every so often, I think: 'What will be with my kids?' We've already lived our lives, in another twenty years we'll be gone. But what will happen to them? Totally no confidence."

Despite my initial impression of Lapid as someone with broad emotionally expressive and operational abilities who guides his family and sets the tone, listening to these sentences left me with the feeling that Lapid carries very weighty emotional baggage with no outlet or relief. Perhaps—as he said—"there's nothing else to grasp onto". I was left wondering how many men like him, though adopting patterns of silently overcoming and continuing to function, suffer from undiagnosed psychic post-trauma reactions, and their raw emotions are transferred to the family in general, including the children.

I was then left with the question of how this unexpressed and non-legitimate anxiety impacts the family relationship.

Expression of emotion is perceived as potentially disruptive during battle, and this is assimilated as part of the masculine character. The fathers' perception that their masculine-paternal role is "to keep their feelings inside" corresponds with the masculine image familiar in Western society and which, in Israeli society, links to the image of the ideal combatant male, influenced by military codes of conduct that require controlling and overcoming feelings (Sasson-Levy, 2006). Accordingly, expressing emotions is perceived as possibly harming sons. In the interviews, in many instances activating one defence mechanism was insufficient for dulling the anxiety, so the fathers activated several defences.

Lapid and Oren noted that their sons suffer from fear. Many children in Israel were fearful during this period, with images of terror attacks filling the newspapers and televisions. But since both Oren and Lapid brought the content of their sons' fears into the interview, and perhaps through them expressed their own fear, the sons may have unconsciously caught their fathers' fear and inability to find an outlet for it and, through projective identification, adopted the fear as their own and expressed it instead of the fathers. If so, it would seem that the fathers' inability of sharing their feelings elsewhere, from a wish to create a sense of safety in their families, in fact transfers the anxiety and fear to the sons under the surface causing anxiety symptoms in the sons.

To sum up: beyond the universal processes undergone by Western society, in the Israeli reality the fathers' silence carries a unique significance. This paternal trait towards sons derives from the emotional stress that Israeli fathers must cope with, and it results in the silencing, in one form or another, of a significant part of their lives and their emotions, thus affecting the developmental stages in their roles as fathers of sons.

So how do fathers behave?

The fathers' gripping emotional conflict that does not allow them to fulfil their traditional role as family protectors while simultaneously being role and identity models for their sons results in paternal behaviours that contradict their statements and encompass conflicting emotional messages. Some fathers encourage mature, masculine, independent behavioural patterns in their sons, stating that it is not good to protect sons, who need to be exposed to the demands of the environment and allowed to bear responsibility for their actions; but their behaviour is actually the reverse. Some declare that the sons need to be protected from any frustration or difficulty and indeed behave that way. Others leave the decision of how far to protect the sons in the mother's control but then express opposition to her ideas. Some express concern that excessive giving to—and giving in to—sons may lead to them being unable to handle difficult situations that arise in the army.

Some educational principles were perceived by the fathers as important in preparing sons for responsibility in general, and functioning in the army in particular. These were generally presented as resistance to mothering statements indicative of indulging anxiety and protecting the sons. Since the fathers were silent during most of the interviews, listening to their voices becomes possible through accurately collecting their statements into one continuous message, which reveals their dynamics.

One obvious example can be found in David's responses. After David and Dina described how their firstborn, a son, misbehaves at school, and his behaviour at home is characterized by dependency, David said: "If he's like he is now when he grows up, he'll also have a problem when he's in the army, for sure!"

Conveying a message to sons that they should conform to the system's requirements expresses an attitude that does not protect the sons but does allow them to feel sure of themselves and internalize the message that the father believes in their ability. David related to the issue of responsibility as important when preparing a son for recruitment:

> "If the child is built right, he finds his place in school, in the army and . . . from there, his future in life. The transition really is sharp.

> He needs to be prepared, you can't keep him wrapped in cotton-wool until he's eighteen and then suddenly throw responsibility at him. Suddenly he'll be there in the army, and there won't be any mother or father who'll . . . wake him and that . . . I did that."

This approach led to David, over the past year, relaxing all his limitations and demands:

> "The closer it comes, you sit less on him . . . when he should go to sleep, and . . . what he's doing . . ."

He shared how hard it is to actually implement this, giving the example of his son's driving licence:

> "Driving, for example. I think, how can it be possible at seventeen to put a car in the hands . . . then you say, ok, in a year he gets . . . a tank, a 150-mm weapon, a submarine, a fighter jet—so you won't give him the car???"

Lapid described a similar behavioural pattern towards his son who was close to recruitment, but his reasons behind this behaviour are different. Lapid wanted his son to enjoy himself as much as possible before recruitment.

> "I . . . for some time now don't say 'no' to the kid on anything . . . anything, even if he angers me. On Sabbath a friend phoned and said, 'Lapid, I just saw your son not driving carefully, you should talk to him.' Two minutes later, he walked in . . . I said, 'Come here, someone just phoned me, said you're not driving carefully.' He answered insolently . . . If that'd happened six months ago, I'd have punished him on the spot: at least two weeks not using the car. Why not now? Because he's getting drafted, and I want to let him enjoy these three months as much as possible."

Later, he explained how this behaviour serves an additional purpose:

> "If you punish him, you make him feel small. On the other hand, because of his recruitment, I let him feel he's allowed to be impudent and express his view, because he's already a personality in his own right . . . a man. I'm afraid of him being a man . . . but . . . you want him to stand on his own two feet, now's the time—what's called, 'fledging'."

Lapid then turned to Leah and continued in the same breath, smiling at her, "Don't cry."

The value of comradeship or sociability appeared in two interviews as important, and in others as part of other topics related to sons being recruited. Eitan, who spoke very little during the interview, primarily voicing his opposition to Ella, who described how she educates their oldest son not to serve in a combat unit, only expressed an unequivocal stance on sociability. On the surface, he didn't link this to his son's future recruitment:

> "For me, it's more important than education . . . social integration and what he gains from the classroom, and how good and pleasant it is for him there, much more than . . . actual learning, because even if he misses a day or two, I don't see that as a huge catastrophe, because he's going to be there eight whole years . . ."

Sefi, however, sees the importance of social acceptance in the context of military service, and his obligation to ready his sons to function in that context:

> "It's important for the child to be involved, socially accepted. Because that's what you also want for his future. The army's a society where . . . you need to know how to cope, with all the tools you've got . . . If you get through childhood well, you should be able to get through the army well."

> "You give the proper tools for the right kind of life. What it is to be decent, to relate to your mate, to respect parents, and . . . that should do the work later. If that doesn't do its job, then, ah . . . somewhere along the line you must have done something wrong. Then he won't do the right thing in the army . . ."

Sefi's statements became increasingly unclear and were left hanging. David also linked friendship to military service:

> "I try to educate to comradeship and giving and contributing and all that. Because in the army you feel it really strongly."

Throughout the world, the majority of fathers educate their sons to values of giving and sociability. In Israel, however, behaviour that superficially seems normative can be accompanied by an "underground" emotional message of profound anxiety over the sons' lives, to the point that, during military service, the son's life might depend on his social skills. The message may be one that the parent is conscious of but does not speak about and is therefore concealed from the son; or it may be unconscious and conveyed with full emotionality, without son or father being aware of what is occurring between them. This example strongly clarifies the statement opening this section: that the same universal, parental behavioural patterns can be imbued with partially conscious or unconscious meaning that is uniquely Israeli.

Fathers who do not release their sons

Not all fathers expressed messages of release relative to their sons, while equipping them with the skills needed to function in the army.

Some fathers showed their difficulty in releasing their sons—some consciously, others not. Boaz said openly:

> "I managed to convince him in some way I'd try to get his military profile lowered . . . I also asked friends in high positions in the army to slot him into a non-combat role but didn't succeed. I don't care that he'll get angry at me—so what?"

Boaz conveyed contradictory messages to his son. The overt message was that he is not willing for his son to serve in a combat unit and will not accept the son's decision to do so. However, unlike the mothers, who intentionally avoid all situations of disagreement with their sons, thus preventing them from creating the distance needed to allow their maturity, Boaz does not seem to have neutralized his son's anger over his manipulations and is actually allowing his son to resist, to choose his own path.

Perhaps this is an effective method of solving the unconscious, impossible paternal conflict: showing open opposition to the son's combat service, Boaz appeases his own internal fears for his son's life and avoids conflict with his wife and being blamed for their son's recruitment into a combat unit, but he also allows his son to mature, to rebel against his life path being chosen for him, and, in the final run, to do as he wanted.

By comparison, Yitzhak's clutching paternal pattern, his difficulty in setting boundaries, parallels the mother's clutching:

> "First of all, I'm disturbed that we p . . . p . . . protect him too much. In truth, our oldest son asks my permission more by way of 'protocol' . . ."

Talking about this obviously allowed Yitzhak to express his ambivalence towards his overprotectiveness towards his sons.

Zak, father of two young sons whose wife, Zehava, is pregnant with their third son, found another trick for preventing his sons from enlisting in combat units:

> "I totally believe that the right direction for the boys is computers, or advanced academic studies . . . there are many professions that aren't combat."

Zak had previously said he expected his sons to be involved in the hi-tech world. Now I wondered whether that statement was linked to his wish to protect his sons in the army, so I asked: "When you talked about hi-tech earlier, were you thinking then about military service?" Zak answered loudly and clearly, "Yes, of course!"

Hillel also commented about sending his sons to a "museum summer camp", rather than a sports-focused camp that develops physical skills, so they won't go into combat units.

A clear definition of the father's place relative to the son's, and their relative roles, allows the son to start shaping his individual masculine identity while adopting parts of the father's image and rejecting others (Benjamin, 1995); similarly, Lewow (2004) stated that

> one of a child's self-needs is to encounter the parents with clear self-boundaries. Only in this way can the child attain direction for her or his own development.

Some fathers tried to void the distance and/or space between themselves and their sons, as though unconsciously driven, like the mothers, by the wish not to allow their sons to undergo the developmental process and, in this way, prevent them from identifying with the image of the masculine warrior. Rafael, who has three young boys, shows this clearly. In childish language he describes how he behaves with his sons and their friends, as though entering a state of mind typical of a child: "I think I'm a different kind of Abba from other daddies. From other fathers."

I smiled and said: "You spoke just now really from the child's perspective."

> Rafael: "That's exactly how I live. That was an excellent example! With the children . . . it's not that I'm becoming child-y . . . but I raise the child to a level where in my view he needs to be; not like other adults, who bring the child down even lower than he is to communicate."

Rafael clarified that this doesn't apply only to his children's friends:

> "I'm familiar with the families in the new township . . . through the children or their dogs . . . I don't know the adults' names, but if they tell me who their child is, I'll know . . . I don't mean 'know' as in 'that's the father of . . .', I mean 'know' at the level of a fist-bump or backslap. There's no just saying 'hello' to each other."

Rafael's body language was excited: with almost every third word, he smacked the sofa. His tone was didactic and conveyed the sense of being pleased and proud of his behaviour. I understood his aggressive, excited body language as expressing other, less pleasant or unequivocal feelings that Rafael unconsciously carries parallel to those of which he is conscious.

Yitzhak also noted using child-like language as demonstrating closeness with his children.

> "I don't select the words I choose with my sons . . . without thinking twice, I can say 'you're fucked up'."

He said the boys tell them almost everything, but the middle son does lie every so often. Yasmin and he called these lies "little bluffs" or "gimmicks"—words for a lovable trait that doesn't require worrying about. I thought that by ignoring the anger and concern aroused nonetheless by the son's lies, they continue to avoid creating distance between them and their son, even though this is possibly what the son wanted to create by lying. Indeed, Yitzhak described his close relationship, lacking hierarchy and distance:

> "We're really not . . . not a 'hurdle' for them . . . they speak to us freely . . . we flow, we don't . . . think too much about it."

The closing statement can be a preconscious expression that Yitzhak's words do, indeed, encode content that he avoids knowing.

Conclusion

Behind the fathers' silence and the few sentences spoken, there is a paternal anxiety over the sons' future enlistment. However, unlike the mothers, who were a "trumpet of anxiety", the fathers tried to neutralize their anxiety with multiple emotional defences: using lower impact language; contradicting statements expressing anxiety immediately after making those statements; relating to worry as an emotionless fact; speaking about anxiety in the feminine gender; using rationalization such as logical reasoning that proves it is not necessary to fear the sons' military service so much; or, alternatively, offering reasons other than fear to direct the sons away from combat service; applying displacement by transferring information from the personal to the general level; or using repression by adopting thoughts that focus on the present.

If the maternal emotional picture does not allow full understanding of the effects on the family of knowledge of a son's future recruitment, then with the fathers we also find only a partial picture. The discussion of the parental couple relationship in chapter four provides a fuller picture of the meaning of parenting boys in Israel.

Notes

1. In the study, every "I-Poem" was transcribed into a numbered listing, with the relevant topic listed alongside. They were prepared separately for mothers and for fathers. The statements were then presented in a table alongside each other, to allow comparison of them. The table also included two "We"-statement columns where the verbs were common to both.

2. *Yediot Aharonot* weekend magazine, "7 Days", 2 April 2004.

3. The main commercial and market centre of the city of Hebron, and a hotbed of violent clashes between Jewish and Muslim residents.

CHAPTER FOUR

Unconscious solution in the couple relationship

> And God said, it is not good for man to be alone, I shall make him [a match opposite][1] him . . .
>
> Genesis 2: 18

> The Sages explain: if he is meritorious, she will match him with worthiness; but if he is not meritorious, she will be oppositional to him to the same measure.
>
> Midrash Rabbah, 17: 3

The couple relationship that transitions into a parental relationship is comprised of latent and overt emotional material residing in the psyches of each partner, including unconscious messages transmitted from earlier generations and further padded out with the unique traits of the specific couple. As a result, it is appropriate to relate to each couple relationship as a separate entity, with its own particular characteristics. To analyse and understand the couple dynamics, it is necessary to distinguish among three separate emotional entities—the two individuals separately, and both linked together as a couple—while acknowledging that, within each individual and in their shared space and link, there are conscious and unconscious processes that are in changing and ongoing reciprocity (Green, 1975; Mann-Shalvi, 2010; Scharff & Scharff, 2011).

Before I had asked the couples about their thoughts and feelings accompanying child-rearing, I expected a range of topics relative to raising children to surface. To my surprise, couples focused primarily on their sons' future recruitment as the conflict in their relationship.

Occasionally harsh exchanges were heard, with a sense of unbridgeable disparity. On other occasions, the tension was a felt presence. Mostly, however, I felt a sense of implicit cooperation between the couple—the converse of conflict and tension. The similarity in the way such vastly different couples expressed this made me feel as though I were attending a cyclical rite. Delving into the parents' words further, I understood that perhaps it was the very conflict between the couple that allowed directing and regulating energy in parental functioning, which, for parents of sons in Israel, is a paradoxical trap, as detailed in chapters two and three.

The depth of the schism in the couple relationships was demonstrated by the table listing "I" statements and "We" statements. I had separated the "I" and "We" words from the interview transcripts, together with the verb following them, and organized these into four columns to enable reviewing the "emotional skeleton" surfacing within them. Two I-sentence columns contained verbs relating to each of the couple, and two We-statement columns contained verbs common to both. I discovered to my surprise that when the parents spoke on general topics connected with raising children, the four columns were full: in other words, couples expressed themselves freely at the individual and jointly shared levels. But once they began talking about their sons' future recruitment, three columns remained empty: only the mothers' I-statement column were full to overflowing; the fathers' remained empty (see chapter three); nor were there any comments shared jointly by the couple. The only thing that Odelia and Oren and David and Dina said in the plural was that they are unable to discuss their sons' future recruitment together—showing the couple-relationship difficulty deriving from this situation.

One couple with no conflict and jointly shared anxiety around their sons' future recruitment was Rafael and Ruth, and their parenting pattern was indeed characterized by overprotectiveness and a sense of unbalanced guilt. The interview with Matan and Mira was the only one where the issue of future recruitment did not surface at all. On checking what differentiated this couple from others, I found that Mira, though born in Israel, had, up until her own recruitment, lived in the United States. As discussed further on, this calls into question whether it is growing up in Israel that is the source of the emotional baggage activated when becoming parents of sons.

The foci of couple tension

Naomi and Noah have a daughter aged four and are expecting a son. Even though he was not born yet, tangible tension could be felt in their relationship regarding his future recruitment. In response to my question about his thoughts and feelings on raising children, Noah immediately said, "I think they'll go into the army". He then tried to repress from his conscious thoughts the danger this represents to his unborn son's life. But Naomi fought with his defences one at a time, until they collapsed, and he "admitted" that yes, in a time of war, his son's life could be endangered:

Noah: "I don't think of the army that much."

Naomi: "Why not, Noah?"

Noah: "Why yes? It's so far ahead."

Naomi: "True, but it *does* exist . . . that's actually a kind of denial of there being an army."

At this point Noah attempted a logical explanation for distancing his threatening thoughts and feelings:

Noah: "So what? He'll go to an old people's home too, at some point."

Naomi: "But in the army, he could die, and in an old-age home . . ."

The three of us laughed at the thought this gave rise to, but Naomi quickly finished the sentence, "you die of good old age". The laughter cut the tension a little but nonetheless left Naomi in the stronger position. The difference between violent death when young and natural death in old age weighted the balance.

Noah tried another argument to convince Naomi that there's no need for concern: "Yesterday you yourself said that getting drunk and driving are more dangerous than the army." But Naomi cut him short: "The army embodies . . . marks the possibility of death!" To this bleak statement, Noah answered sharply: "It does not!"

As though alarmed at the escalation in the discussion, Noah asked if that was what she really thought. Naomi responded: "Only if he will go into a brigade . . . something like Intelligence or clerical, then no, not, but if he's going into some elite unit, then there's the possibility he could be killed."

Interestingly, when speaking of the possibility of non-combatant recruitment, which calms her anxiety, Naomi used the future tense, but for commando service she switched to the present, as though the fetus she carries is about to enter the army any second.

Noah tried to calm her with facts: "More soldiers get killed on their way to and from home."

Naomi answered impatiently: "Yes, Noah, but for me it's something that increases the danger . . . Look, it's hard to know right now if there'll be wars or not, but in war it's obvious there's the possibility of dying!" This statement collapsed Noah's last stand. He withdrew into himself, leaving Naomi with her anxiety as he whispered to himself:

"War really is something risky."

Their relationship was tense from the start, manifested in arguments in many areas—education, city- or farm-based living, the name of their child, their different attitudes towards boys and girls, and more. Usually Naomi went silent, but on the matter of future recruitment she persisted and she spoke repeatedly of the dangers this son in her womb may have to face, her tone charged with anxiety mingled with anger, insistent until her husband reached the "yes, dear" moment.

The question then is: when it came to her anxiety over her son's life, did she feel justified in standing up for her views, finding an object for aggression accumulated in her which she cast at Noah during other couple-relationship conflicts?

Since it seems as though all parents of boys in Israel are caught in an insoluble conflict that locks down their parental functioning (as detailed previously), charged energy from the parental system is directed at and onto the couple relationship and vice versa.

On the one hand, Noah and Naomi's parental conflict added to the tension in the couple relationship; on the other, it also served as an aperture through which accumulated aggressive energy, especially in Naomi, could find release. This is not a value statement of "good or bad for the couple relationship" but an observation describing the existing interpersonal dynamic at the foundation of the conflictual interaction. The question of whether it helps the couple to survive their couple relationship or breaks it up depends on many other personality factors in each couple, which would require further information.

The way Yasmin and Yitzhak coped with the issue was different. Yasmin shared her anxiety over her sons' lives during military service while Yitzhak was out of the room, then added: "Maybe he'll be a Shekemist? It'd be nicer for me . . . no, actually I'd die of shame."

I reflected: "It's a conflict of sorts . . ." to which Yasmin responded: "It's a tough, conflict because you don't want anything to happen to your kids; not even when protecting the country you love so much."

Yitzhak returned and reacted sharply: "What do you mean, sacrifice . . . that's idiotic . . . a human sacrifice, that's rubbish . . ."

Yasmin looked at him, stunned. It seemed that she could no longer bear the emotional significance that Yitzhak applied to her words, and she tried to link them to him. They began "tossing" between them ownership of the harsh feelings roused by the conflict.

> Yasmin: "It's not me that said that, you don't want anything to happen to your children."
>
> Yitzhak: "If you knew one of the children would die in the army . . . tomorrow you'd . . . if it was a hundred percent for sure, you wouldn't stay ten minutes."
>
> Yasmin: "Of course! It's a conflict of sorts, but . . . if he became a Shekemist or a clerk of some kind . . . you'd die of shame . . ."

Yasmin's remark to Yitzhak that "you don't want anything to happen to your children" cast him in the role of protector and guardian of the sons. But Yitzhak returned that role to her by saying, three times, "you would". Yasmin tried to contain the conflict with, "It's a conflict of sorts". But a force of which she was unaware caused her to retreat into the typical couple relationship's division of roles as she cast the responsibility for her son being a commando onto Yitzhak: "If he would become a Shekemist . . . you'd die of shame." Yitzhak was unable to take on a role that allowed his sons to adopt the Israeli masculine identity together with blame for endangering their lives, and he reacted furiously, tossing the blame onto her for wanting a commando son:

> "Shame? That's not part of the equation . . . shame? What's the connection with shame? What do you care what others think of you?"

His reaction left Yasmin no choice but to fill both roles simultaneously: that of the protector and guardian, and that of nurturing and encouraging the Israeli masculine warrior identity.

> "Of course I don't care what others think of me, I'd die to think that was my son, that . . ."

Possibly for the first time, she spoke from the depths of her soul, in an unaccustomed way:

> ". . . that he's not a fighter, that he's not doing that . . . that he isn't training, that he isn't progressing, that . . ."

She thought for a moment, smiled, and grimaced:

> "Yes, progressing . . . not . . . quickly enough."

Then she burst into embarrassed laughter, as if to say "Caught with my guard down: I'm trying to say something, but as a mother I'm not permitted to, so instead, I've managed to tiptoe between the raindrops." The sense of helplessness persisted in the room, together with a feeling of potential change.

The couple seemed to have difficulty preserving good relations with the ongoing conflict over their son's future life-endangering army service. The tension creates a feeling of disparity that cannot be bridged, penetrating from the parental to the couple level.

With some couples, my presence and the interview created an opportunity to express weighty feelings. Instead of polemics around "who holds the truth", an opportunity arose for the couple to acknowledge their opposing stances, shaping a new couple-relationship space in which they could express personal thoughts and feelings. In these situations, the tension dropped, and separation formed between disputes at the parental level and the couple relationship, enabling space to understand and support constructive criticism.

Eitan and Ella argued strongly, with a feeling of hostility and tension, about the correct messages to convey to their eldest son, relative to his future recruitment. Generally, Ella spoke loudly and quickly, expressing herself articulately, unequivocally, and expansively, whereas Eitan was silent. With what sounded like a mix of anxiety, anger, and helplessness, she presented her views opposing their son's recruitment. She was angry with the army, with the Israeli reality, and with Eitan, too, whom she may unconsciously have identified as the representative of this reality, including the army. Prominently felt was the sense that this issue brings turbidity into the couple relationship.

But when Ella and Eitan could acknowledge the conflict as part of their parenthood, their tone of speech relaxed, as though the tension had dissipated. As Ella described:

> "My oldest son has American citizenship. I often tell him to go and study overseas rather than enlist. But Eitan *really* doesn't like when I say that. He doesn't belong to the state, this child, nor to the army. He belongs to me and my husband and himself. And I don't trust this army."

Eitan disagreed with her:

> "I don't agree with what she thinks about the army . . . that they don't benefit from being in it. My experience of the army is completely different . . . it's not an issue that causes me stress . . . but she has [him for] more hours than I do."

Thus, although an emotionally charged conflict took place between them at the superficial level, a cooperative discourse began based in the couple-relationship space where the parental conflict could exist. In acknowledging each other's complex stances, the existence of conflicting messages necessary for full functioning as parents of the son is allowed: Ella voiced protectiveness towards her son's life; Eitan voiced encouragement of the son's independence and maturation while adopting values of military service without fear of being silenced. When Ella acknowledged Eitan's opposition to her views, she actually acknowledged his perception; when Eitan acknowledged his inferiority because of the limited time during which he could convey his message, he allowed her the space to fulfil her protective role. In this way their son receives all the messages he needs for maturing from parents functioning as a parental unit, something each parent singly would not be able to fully provide.

As for Yasmin and Yitzhak, they seemed initially to present a shared outlook characterized by overprotectiveness of their sons while simultaneously educating them to volunteerism during military service. But a second look discloses an inverse emotional picture.

Yasmin presented her educational views expansively, with great praise of the children, while Yitzhak remained silent. I felt that she related to them with some idealization—part of the parenting pattern characterized by the overprotectiveness that, both said, typified their parenting. I also felt that, through his silence, Yitzhak was expressing unspoken opposition. I wondered if acknowledgement of the existence of conflicts between them was not allowed.

Towards the end of the interview, in fact, a deep conflict between Yasmin and Yitzhak burst into the open. It was lengthy; I present only parts of it here.

Initially, Yasmin appeared to be interested in Yitzhak's intention, completing his sentences, so her sudden resistance came across as explosive—as though she couldn't contain herself any longer:

> Yitzhak: "Look, the first thing that bothers me is that we . . . 'protect' them too much."

Yasmin: "That we're a protective family?"

Yitzhak: "Too much, yes. And we send them to schools that are, so called . . ."

He and Yasmin completed this sentence together:

"Elitist. As far as population, no violence, and also no . . ."

So far, Yasmin had joined in with Yitzhak, but slowly I felt her becoming stressed as Yitzhak continued:

"Their immediate environment and our closest friends are from the same . . . background. The question is: what will be??? After all, at some point they'll come face to face with the real world . . . for example, in the army. I'm this good little boy from . . . an arts school in Haifa, and here I am, joining Golani . . . there's a whole mix of people from all layers . . . all types of behaviour . . . At first I was in shock, it wasn't normal . . . in the end I loved it, and . . . the question is how they'll withstand the pressure if they come from that kind of place. I'd like them to be able to cope in that situation."

Yasmin's body language began to disclose emotions than had not been discerned until now. When Yitzhak continued:

"We're always on top of them, and preventing them from getting to that, and I think it's worth them getting to that. Because . . . I . . . they don't live in a bubble.. and li . . ."

Yasmin cut him short sharply and defiantly burst into his statement:

"Why do you think that they don't get to coping with the real world?? Because they're in slightly better schools . . . so what??"

I felt she was getting pressured and defensive. It is not clear whether it was being aware of recruitment-related anxiety that caused the pressure or whether something is deficient with their children's education. Yasmin said:

"But look, these are our friends whom we chose, it's . . . it's not as though we were forced to be friends with them . . . those who are suited to us . . ."

A heated argument continued between them for some minutes. It was harsh, with no listening, in the guise of a cultural discussion. Yasmin veered between insult and sarcastic, angry defiance. They repeated their stances with no common ground between them. Yasmin was insistent:

"I don't think we envelop them too much. On the contrary, I think it's worth them having as many good experiences as possible, rather than as many experiences of . . ."

But Yitzhak repeated his statement incessantly:

"We protect them . . . we protect them too much."

Suddenly, Yasmin expressed her stress:

"I don't know . . . I don't feel good with this, it doesn't speak to me . . ."

In one instant, a change had occurred. She turned towards me, raising her voice and adopting Yitzhak's approach:

"Look, it can be that it's sometimes necessary to struggle . . . one of the things Yitzhak's always saying is that I see the children's problems too clearly. I mean, I'm onto them before anyone else is, and sometimes he says that I invent problems for them. Afterwards it turns out to be true. Then he gets even madder at me for finding them."

Her closing words were accompanied by laughter. As with Ella and Eitan, the moment the conflict was put into words, Yasmin showed relief and greater ease through liberating laughter. It seems that when Yasmin doesn't allow herself to acknowledge the conflict between them and tries to align with Yitzhak's views, which do not accord with her own, the tension builds insider her until she can no longer contain it: it breaks through, confusing her and causing her to switch stances suddenly. But, once a clear division of roles between them was achieved and each mutually acknowledged the existence of the conflict, calm ensued.

Odelia and Oren described their inability to reach an understanding, let alone agreement, on how to raise their sons relative to anxiety over the boys' lives when they enlist. These latest insights allow us to see that once they could acknowledge their inability to function as a couple on this issue, they could sustain a relationship of evident mutual listening and acceptance, gentle speech, and an overall calm atmosphere, as each presented and represented an emotional and ideological view of the other.

For example, Odelia said:

"Oren and I used to argue about it a lot. I'd say that when the kids grow up, around fourteen, fifteen, we'd leave the country. And

> Oren would say: Ok, I'll send you postcards . . . It's, like, a subject we can't talk about, and our communication is still developing."

She spoke slowly, loudly, emphasizing each word by slapping her knee:

> "They'll get to be eighteen. Now we're at . . . an understanding that we simply can't discuss this."

Several times towards the end of the interview they brought up the conflicts between them. Odelia said:

> "Perhaps, by contrast with what I said earlier, that we just argue about it, now we really understand that we just can't talk about it."

And Oren followed up:

> "Yes, hmmm, I think we have very different opinions on this. Odelia says that we should leave, and I say, OK, I'll send you postcards . . ."

Later, he summarizes:

> "I can . . . it's true that . . . there's tension between two oppositional directions. Two completely different stances."

Laughter, which often appeared in interviews once the existence of the conflict was acknowledged, often functions as shared release (Levi, 2004). Laughter can be understood as relief felt by a couple during discussions where, by acknowledging the disparity between them, a couple-relationship space is established which, instead of a frozen relationship, allows for discourse that expresses opposing opinions while simultaneously allowing them to function as parents.

We have seen that Israel parenting to boys traps parents in ways that make it difficult for them to function. The tension derived from the internal conflict seems to be released through argument and directed to their couple relationship, placing continuous pressure on it. However, when a space is created that allows them to acknowledge that conflict exists between them, it allows containing and filling the contradictory parental tasks. But if parents blur the conflict between them, then their couple relationship fills with unclear, hostile, stressful content that will find alternative ways of releasing itself.

Lost guilt feelings

The feelings about raising sons and acknowledging their future recruitment appeared directly and clearly among the fathers and mothers. Guilt feelings, however, appeared in a different way—at the level of the couple relationship, their existence shown in behavioural patterns characterized by overprotectiveness of sons and compensation, and through the mothers' attacks on the fathers' masculinity. Puzzlingly, when mothers did not initiate putting blame on the fathers, the fathers did so themselves: "Do you remember telling me I'd be responsible if he goes to commandos?" Such statements initiated the maternal blaming that appeared in different variations, signifying that the father is responsible for endangering the son's life in the army.

Several relationship patterns developed from this point. The wife would continue attacking the father's masculinity, causing him to become defensive, with conflict developing between them. Interestingly, the men did not attack the mothers' femininity. These arguments usually ended with the fathers falling silent, taking on the blame and containing it for the sake of the couple unit as a whole. Odelia, for example, casts blame on Oren:

> "Oren was in the standing army for several years . . . His service period was really important to him. He's very proud of it, and the boys catch on to that and really want to mimic Oren . . . Once I got really angry at Oren because he told the kids he was a commander in the army. I don't want them to be anything in the army. For Oren it's really . . . a positive experience. It took me a long time to accept that. I was in the army during the Lebanon War, and . . . for me it's all linked with . . . you know . . . death. I don't see the army as a positive experience."

As long as Odelia acknowledged the legitimacy of Oren's emotional stance and her own difficulty in accepting it, Oren did not dispute her, despite the harsh blame contained in her words. But when she added that the boys are afraid of being killed but can't tell him because they fear he expects them to be as strong and heroic as he, Oren had difficulty in accepting this and in a weak voice tried to defend himself: "Uri did raise that with me!"

The firstborn son of another couple, Dina and David, whose relationship is clearly characterized by love and mutual respect, was being drafted in about a month. Dina was the main speaker throughout, careful not to hurt David. Unlike other mothers, it was she who shared the guilt feelings that accompany her mothering of sons:

> "I'm afraid that *if anything happens to him, I'll go crazy thinking that I directed him towards it* . . . latterly I've also been telling myself a different narrative. That if I . . . even if I say nothing, something could

happen (he could be killed) and I'll say afterwards, why didn't I tell him to go . . ."

I asked: "Is there no escaping the guilt?" She responded: "Not for me . . . I imagine with some others too."

David looked at her and gave a small smile. Until now, he had handed the role of speaker to Dina, but he suddenly changed his position, cut in, and started to release her from the guilt feelings by taking them on himself. He declared:

"I constantly try to neutralize that in her . . ."

Instantly, Dina responded with what I experienced as relief, compared to her manner when describing her own guilt feelings: she slowly started to blame David as responsible for his wish that their son enlist for commando service.

"You spoke about the army in the negative sense, 'If you're not . . . then how will you manage in the army . . .' and I didn't like that."

She pounded the air with her left hand. Not only did David not become defensive, but quite the opposite: acknowledging the couple-relationship space that contains the conflict, he took clear responsibility for the blame levelled at him:

"We don't agree on this issue. She, of course, always said it's not okay that I throw him into the army."

I thought that "of course" corresponds to the understanding that he adopts the blame for possible harm to their son as an unconscious resolution for the parental stress in which they are interlocked. When I repeated, "throwing him into the army?", Dina reacted strongly, "Yes, yes!" Her response to the very imprecise way I repeated David's statement clarified that talking about it eased things for her. From this point on, David and Dina did remain in their roles on each side of the dispute, but David's opposition was minor: it was apparent that he was ready to accept the blame and contain the guilt for any harm to their son in the army.

It seems that Dina did not feel relief: her attack on David became even harsher:

"When the recruitment order came . . . it made me very frightened, but you were proud . . . what they now call 'poisoned',[2] . . . when I first met him, he wasn't like that, but I think he is now."

Dina spoke as though she was even disowning her own responsibility for having chosen him:

> "And then there's the guys from the army, with all their army stories . . . it's a dominant topic. And I think that anything our son chooses that isn't . . . a combat unit, would be a kind of disappointment for David. I was afraid that . . . it'd be projected in some kind of way on the boys, and they'd be forced to do something in order not to . . . disappoint, and then . . . they'd go . . ."

I asked, "How did that manifest between you?" David answered: "Sometimes she asked me not to mention the army, at least not only in . . ."

His voice faded out; Dina clarified, cynically, that she has no problem talking to her sons about her non-combat service, since no danger is involved in her descriptions—it is David whose military service and "poisoned" status constitute the danger to their sons' lives. With that, David took the blame on himself, and the responsibility if their son fulfilled the father's expectations and became a commando; but he indicated how difficult that was for him: "She's right that if they do it only to please me, then it's really harsh . . ."

Dina ignored his feelings and carried on: "I'm a bit afraid of that, they'll think they're not fulfilling his expectations, in their studies[3] and as commandos, for example."

Beyond the harsh content, it is hard to ignore Dina's sadness when she notes just how clear David's expectations of his sons are. David's consent is also sad and touching. This is a couple who, against their wishes, are helpless when faced with this dynamic. In content, Dina blamed David, and David accepted the blame; but in their body language there is no blaming, no guilty parties—just two hurting, scared, sad parents.

From Dina's point of view, David's entire masculine identity poses a threat to the lives of her sons in a way of which she is not conscious, arousing her need to force a wedge between them:

> "I think you'll be disappointed if a child of yours doesn't go for commando service . . ."

David tried to find a reason that would legitimize a son not enlisting for combat service:

> "I can accept it if there's a reason, some medical or other reason . . ."

But Dina was at the ready:

> "I mean without a reason, simply because he doesn't want to enlist, like that pacifist friend of his."

David again releases Dina from responsibility but doesn't retreat, allowing himself to authentically express himself as an Israeli male and father, containing the conflict. Quietly and sadly, he said: "Yes, that would bother me a lot . . . and that he's even connected with someone like that."

As detailed in chapter three, later David expressed concern about telling his son about his military past, unsure whether it would cause his son to fear military service, adding that he doesn't know whether it's even possible to prepare someone for something so tough. Perhaps that is what caused Dina, towards the interview's end, again to put the blame on David: "I'm always thinking about how he'll react, if his son would want to evade . . . don't know . . ."

And David agreed with her: "Yes, it would be very difficult for me, I don't know how I'd feel . . . how I'd attack it, I'm sure . . . I'd also see it as . . . a kind of failure on my part."

Rather than leaving David as the only one carrying guilt for endangering their sons' lives, I suggested a softer possibility, in the form of a conflict: "So it truly is a conflict?" and David answered, "Conflict, yes, yes."

Maternal attack on the masculine combat identity of fathers, casting blame for potentially endangering their boys' lives, is also shown in Leah and Lapid's relationship.

Leah and Lapid seemed satisfied with their couple relationship; this was evident through their affectionate body language and expressions of affection, admiration, warmth, and mutual respect. One would therefore not expect any harsh emotional or ideological conflict between them. However, once the topic of raising sons came up, with its accompanying anxiety regarding future recruitment, serious conflict appeared, expressed in extreme phraseology that matched the division of roles encountered in other couples.

Lapid expressed a wish to serve as an identity model for his sons:

> "I knew I was going to enlist, I did the army, I did reserve duty, I volunteered for reserve duty after my injury, and that's how I educated my children . . . that you go into the army. Of course, it can't be any other way."

Leah burst into his sentence:

> "I'm the *opposite!* Even when Rabin was still there . . . I said to Lapid, 'No!' Even before our son gets his first call-up papers, I don't want to be here."

The conflict recurred several times, emphasizing their oppositional views but accompanied by mutual respect and understanding. Lapid said:

> *"I'm exactly the opposite,* I'm attached . . ."

and again Leah interrupted and continued with her own view:

> "I really don't want it, don't want it."

Lapid countered with:

> "I'm attached to this country, but I also have periods of rumination."

Leah looked at him, and in a defiant tone, said:

> "I'm also attached to this country."

Whenever Lapid expressed doubts about raising his children in Israel, Leah confronted him with the fact that she still wants to leave the country and that if their son were killed, Lapid would be responsible—as if saying to him: "This is my role as mother, to counteract." It was clear that from the moment the first call-up papers arrived their son would be considered a deserter if he left the country, but neither of them said this outright. Another example demonstrates the argument:

> Lapid: "The boundary between . . . frontlines and home front have blurred. Because, looking back, I think more civilians were killed than soldiers.[4] So it's scary to raise kids here."

From this point on, they interrupted each other frequently, or spoke simultaneously:

> Leah: "So . . . there's no reason to be here."
>
> Lapid: "No. There's no reason for us to be somewhere else, I'm not capable of living in some other country when I know that the policeman on the corner isn't one of my own."
>
> Leah: "So what? I know I'm with my family, with my kids, and everyone's whole and healthy."

Lapid: "No. We've got to cope, eject the enemy . . ."

Leah: "No . . . not with my flesh . . . my kids and family are what interests me."

Lapid: "So, listen. This generation will fight, and the next, and I hope that eventually there'll . . . there'll be . . . peace . . . That's how it is."

That's when Leah said, quietly:

> "I don't want to be here. We've got no choice."

What is special about Leah and Lapid, in my view, is the conscious way they defined the division of roles between them, and their emotional openness. Their repetition, in different formulations, of the same statement suggests that in addition to coping with the present, their—unconscious—goal is to ready the emotional infrastructure for a future bereavement. Leah shared her current approach—one that exempts her from feelings of guilt in the future—when she described how she lets Lapid decide what to allow or prohibit, so that if something happens to their sons, he will be accountable:

> "I can say 'no' to the boys, and Lapid plays at being considerate, but he has the . . . the final word. I also ask Lapid about everything: 'What do you think? Yes or no?'"

I asked: "Do you use Lapid?" Leah answered: "Always." I asked: "Otherwise, you'll only say 'no'?" Lapid answered very decisively: "That's true, what you say, it's exactly like that."

I heard relief in Lapid's voice over my identifying the fact that Leah "uses" him, but Leah didn't react to the stress showing in his reaction:

> "It's very convenient for me to rely on his views, on what he decides."

I prompted: "Because . . .", and Leah answered:

> "As he says to me: 'You're playing small-minded.' That's how I am, I enjoy it."

I asked why she found that comfortable; she answered:

> "Because I depend on him for everything, and it's great."

I became insistent: "But what does this behaviour support? What are your released from?" Leah answered in an "isn't it obvious" tone:

> "From responsibility. Afterwards . . . I can come to him with complaints. He knows that."

Leah's closing remarks confirm that indeed she and Lapid share a coordinated emotional dynamic that addresses both their needs, as witnessed by Lapid describing that he must conceal his fears and weaknesses from Leah and the children because otherwise he'll cause them greater insecurity.

The feminine attack on the father's commando masculinity

We have observed how mothers attack the fathers' masculine identity because, to them, sons' identification with their fathers potentially endangers their sons' lives. How does this actually occur?

Mothers adopted a dominant stance in all areas related to raising their sons, while silencing their fathers' voices. Sometimes they attacked the fathers' absence of masculinity through mockery, sometimes their attack was aimed at content at the very base of masculinity, and sometimes their attack contained blame for the possible future death of a son.

This was Naomi's stance when Noah said that the only time he felt he'd done something of value was during his military service:

> "I know there are homes where, from the start, the kids are suckled on 'what you'll do in the army'. You hear it: the father was in this or that unit . . . and the grandfather was in that other unit . . . But with us, there's no such danger . . ."

Naomi laughed briefly and, from that point on, mocked Noah for not being a strong Israeli male—clarifying that if he were, she would fight him:

> "Let's say our son asked: 'Abba, what did you do in the army?' The way I know Noah, he wouldn't be able to say . . ."

Then she lowered her voice, mimicking a "tough guy":

> "Ah.. we took this.. and we went there . . . and we were in this unit . . ."

Noah cut in:

> "Because I didn't . . ."

But Naomi ignored him and carried on:

"Like Bibi, who said they almost froze along the way, and he's got these stories about 'The Unit'.[5] It wouldn't be of value here, Noah won't tell how he raised the turret and how . . ."

Naomi burst out laughing, making a circular movement with her hand as though inserting something into a round aperture:

". . . he oiled the tank."

She used movements possibly suggestive of a sexual nature. Noah tried to oppose:

"He won't ask about that, it's not interesting."

But Naomi was insistent:

"Why . . . he'll ask, 'What do you do with this, and that . . .?'"

Noah continued defending himself against a message that blames him for the possible death of their unborn son by disdaining himself as a non-combatant male: "True, I don't have a story of heroism."

Naomi closed this with:

"It could be that if Noah was like that, then I'd have to be concerned about restraining it, but . . . there won't be any need . . . if Noah was one of those that think 'I'm taking my son from the moment he's three and make him run, play football', as though it's clear he's got this 'little buddy' . . . I think I'd have to restrain that . . . because I'm worried his head would be full of, football, cars . . . And then he'll go into the army or something . . ."

From couple relationship to parenthood and back

As detailed previously, mothers and fathers found themselves trapped in a conflict that is unresolvable, difficult to contain, and derived from the fact that despite social changes in the masculine image in the Western world and in Israel, there is still a great degree of identification between the ideal masculine image and the commando soldier. Therefore, if the parents allow their sons to adopt Israeli masculine identity, they are essentially allowing them to enlist as combat soldiers and possibly risk their lives. Parents who deflect sons from undergoing these developmental stages are sabotaging their sons' separation–individuation.

It is too easy within this stress-ridden dynamic to take sides with one or the other parent. Observing the situation through the concept of concealed division of roles between the couple therefore allows analysing and thinking about their shared and separate processes.

In the context of being parents to sons in Israel, holding opposing roles simultaneously—containing loss anxiety while allowing them to adopt a masculine identity that entails military service and possible death—blame and guilt must also be contained, and the sense of helplessness that is simultaneously aroused must be coped with.

This stress from the parental arena transfers to the couple-relationship level—it may be easier to cope with a conflict expressed through the relationship than with a psychic conflict that locks down parenting. In actuality, an agreement exists between the father and the mother, through the unconscious mutual mechanism of projective identification—splitting off one part of the self that is in conflict with another and projecting it onto the other (Klein, 1946), thereby transforming intrasubjective conflict into an intersubjective one—thus partitioning the anxiety and blame over the sons between them. Thus, by perpetuating the tension between them, the couple cooperate in containing it: ingeniously and unconsciously, it is precisely through the conflict itself that they allow their sons to receive all the parenting functions.

Significant theoretical developments in the field of unconscious processes operating between the couple and within the family convey an understanding of the couple and parental processes revealed in this study. Dicks (1967), for example, viewed marriage as an ongoing state of processes of projective identification and mutual internalization. He claimed that the couple's interactions can be understood in terms of the conscious needs of each partner, together with unconscious shared assumptions and agreements. The same dynamic also occurs unconsciously in parental relationships with children, couples, and families (Scharff & Scharff, 2014).

The following metaphor demonstrates how the parents cope with this situation. Imagine a bowl representing the parents' shared space, into which the parenting tasks are poured. Mothers pour in the need to protect their sons, expressing anxiety over their lives, helplessness over the inability to prevent their recruitment, and guilt over not being able to protect them while, simultaneously, cooperating in educating their sons to values that may eventually bring them to enlisting as commandos—as well as, at a deeper emotional level, guilt over their libidinal attraction to their sons. They also empty into the bowl their need to gradually release their sons so that the latter can adopt their separate masculine identity. Fathers pour into this bowl their role as protectors, loss anxiety, and the helplessness that fills them too, especially unbearable guilt because, being Israeli males, they may risk their sons' lives—a guilt also intensified at the unconscious level by the paternal wish for the sons' deaths.

In a second phase, parents redivide the conflictual tasks between them, such that they do not coexist in that same parent, preventing the parent from fulfilling the parental task.

The maternal conflict, involving an almost symbiotic connection with the son compared to the need to release him, had the mothers leaving themselves in the role of guardian of their sons' lives by keeping them close at hand, while also fighting their sons' assumption of a commando identity. Mothers also held on to the function of containing and expressing the emotions of loss anxiety and helplessness.

With their silence, fathers allow the mothers to do this, providing an outlet for those same feelings that the fathers also experience. Fathers occasionally attempted, weakly, to resist the mothers, thereby allowing for the existence of a voice—for the mothers, too—that opens an avenue that allows the sons to adopt a masculine identity. The primary function of the fathers, however, is to contain the guilt feelings that the mothers cannot take upon themselves. Regarding these guilt feelings, the meaning of the couple's role division seems more complex. The objective of unconscious cooperation between the parents is to exempt themselves from containing the conflict individually; had the fathers contained the guilt feelings themselves, they would not experience any relief. Perhaps this is why, when mothers did *not* blame fathers, the latter still took the blame on themselves, as a reminder that segued into close detailing by the mother of the future guilt to be borne by the father should the son be harmed.

An additional type of cooperation occurs in this exchange of parental tasks: to release the fathers of the psychic burden involved in carrying the guilt feelings as an internal conflict, the mothers adopted the role of blaming the fathers, and only then were the fathers able to take on responsibility for this blame. In this way, in one move, the mothers exempted themselves from guilt and were fully free to play their role of protector, guardian, and the one who voices the loss anxiety and helplessness. The fathers, for their part, were exempted from the need to contain the conflict within themselves of both blaming themselves and containing the guilt. When blame came from the mothers, the conflict was externalized between the father and mother and did not exist within the father's psyche.

Although it is not easy to be blamed for causing future harm to a son's life, it is apparently more bearable when that allows wives to fill their roles as the protector who is concerned about, and expresses, the anxiety. Additionally, bringing the conflict into the interpersonal space allows fathers to take the upper hand with the mothers occasionally, thereby resisting the feeling of guilt, experiencing some relief from the weight of carrying the emotional baggage, and representing the need to allow the son to mature and consolidate a separate masculine identity.

This couple dynamic can also be understood as psychic preparation by the parents for the situation that causes their anxiety. In the interviews, statements were reiterated relating to a state of mourning over fallen sons. In this way, they readied themselves for the worst by splitting—instead of each separately needing to contain the tremendous bereavement together with guilt feelings, a combination that could cause the collapse of them both. The husband continues to be charged with the role of being strong and supporting the wife, who expresses the pain and mourning for them both and receives the support that will help her prevent collapse. Together, they can contain the painful, even torturous feelings, allowing them to continue living and functioning as parents for their other children.

Through this sophisticated unconscious relationship, the couples cooperate in finding a solution to being trapped in the paternal and maternal conflict that allows neither of them to fulfil their roles, enabling them to give their son the range of parenting functions that he needs to grow and mature.

Couples with a steadfast relationship were able to contain the stress and burden of parenthood and preserve a balance in their relationship; for those with a relationship rife with conflict, the stress was an outlet for dispute and release of the already tense emotional baggage.

An ancient masculine commando identity

One of the earliest couples in the Scriptures coping with the issue of masculine commando identity are Rebecca and Isaac, whose conflict centres on their sons Esau and Jacob. Isaac sides with the son who has adopted the hunter-warrior identity, Rebecca with the son who "sits in the tents" close at hand. This is paralleled in the myth narratives and in Freud's dream. These and the other examples indicate that the division of roles typical of Israeli mothers and fathers does indeed exist in states where parents find themselves coping, from the start of their sons' lives, with threat to these sons' lives—a threat that is inseparable from their masculine identities and therefore from their processes of maturation.

We find a parallel dynamic operating at the national level. An organization named "Four Mothers"[6]—which despite its name included fathers—called for the IDF's withdrawal from Lebanon with a slogan that did not mention soldiers or army but called on "taking our boys out of Lebanon". During the disengagement period from the Gaza Strip, another organization, called "Shuvi: The Soldiers' Mothers",[7] called on the prime minister in the following words:

> To the Prime Minister. Sir, guard our sons. As mothers, we raised our sons to serve in the IDF and take part in protecting the State of Israel. . . .

It closes with an additional approach:

> Thousands of mothers have already signed.

In this organization, too, numerous men were registered.[8] A sticker also made its appearance with the slogan, "War is not my language" and signed off by "The Fifth Mother".

Notes

1. The accepted English translation, "helpmeet", is far from precise. The two Hebrew words actually mean something more like "equal" and "against", hence the translation here.
2. Slang for a commando whose identification with combat service and the military is total, enthusiastic, and devoid of criticism.
3. Of science-based subjects including mathematics, as opposed to those studying arts/humanities and whom Dina may see as more emotionally connected and therefore less likely to continue on to masculine combat behaviour.
4. A reference to suicide bombings that had caused over 1,500 deaths and over 9,000 injuries.
5. "The Unit" refers to one of the elite commando units in which current Israeli Prime Minister Benjamin Netanyahu served. It undertakes dangerous, complex operations, and acceptance into it involves an extremely rigorous selection process.
6. Following Judaic tradition of the four founding mothers, Sarah, Rebecca, Rachel, and Leah.
7. *Shuvi*: Hebrew, singular, feminine, imperative: meaning "return".
8. An example of such a notice can be found in *Ha'aretz*, 20 July 2005, p. 5 (www.shuvi.org).

CHAPTER FIVE

Parenting from Holocaust to heroism

> Remember what Amalek did to you on your journey out of Egypt, how they surprised you on the road and cut off all the weak people at your rear, when you were parched and weary. . . .
>
> Deut. 25: 17–19

In Israel, parenthood with sons and couple-relationship patterns with their accompanying emotional worlds are formed in reaction to the unconscious entrapment between oppositional parenting tasks. The emotions aroused through awareness of a son's future recruitment also arise from the powerful unconscious emotional processes echoing myths and Biblical narratives such as the Binding of Isaac (Guvrin, 1935). They chiefly revolve around aggressive potential and libidinal charges within the human psyche, and also directed towards children.

Another significant component in the emotional makeup of parents of sons in Israel is not easy to write about, and possibly equally not easy to read about—namely, the way that the Holocaust experience, focal to the collective Israeli identity and memory (Segev, 1991), interferes with parenting in the context of sons enlisting for military service.

We can relate to insights arising in this regard as observation of the type that Deleuze called "rezoom" (Deleuze & Guattari, 1975). This does not limit itself to causal search but, rather, allows multidimensional, multivalent thinking comprised of a system of interconnections that do not organize around one centre but can add on insights by acknowledging that it is impossible to fully realize "that which cannot be comprised, found across the surface of being" (Luski, 2001, p. 14).

Through my clinical work, and through meetings between "Holocaust second-generation Israelis and Jews and second-generation Germans", I became aware of how the personal and national Holocaust history penetrates the hearts of the second and third generations, manifesting in diverse patterns that have no direct contact with the Holocaust at the personal level, the national level, or even the international level, including in Israel–German relations (Mann-Shalvi, 2007a).

When conducting the interviews, however, even I was affected by a "blind spot" with regard to the powerful connection, at the personal and familial levels, between the Holocaust and IDF. Parents were not asked for biographical details concerning their own parents, so I would have no idea which of my interviewees were children of Holocaust survivors. The Holocaust appeared explicitly in only three couples in a single, and somewhat laconic, manner: in two interviews with a mention that the interviewees' parents were Holocaust survivors, as Gabi, pregnant for the first time, noted:

> "I look at the place I come from, and where my mother comes from. My mother comes from having no family, she's a 'light' Holocaust survivor,[1] she came from the Czechoslovak Republic with her mother, but her father was left there . . . The grandmother still lives, but we hardly know her. I visited her for the first time three years ago, I think, but there's no connection, that's to say . . . I got from my mother things that she had no one to get them from . . . she learned everything herself. And the way she's involved with me now that I'm pregnant . . . it's a different starting point."

Dina said:

> "Our family looks to me, all in all, like a pretty average Israeli family, Zionist, *tzabars*[2] . . . In the previous generation, my parents are Holocaust survivors, but not David's. That is, they are to some extent, they fled, really, right before the Holocaust . . ."

In the interview with Ruth, mother of three sons, the Holocaust appeared in a somewhat puzzling manner when Ruth tried to clarify the difference between conversation with her boys or with girls:

> "I don't know what it is to raise girls, because I have three boys. But I can sense them. For example, when we go out for a day trip, our friends' daughters like to travel with us . . . and suddenly with the girls a discussion about the Holocaust came up. With my boys it's 'yes' 'no' . . ."

Ruth explained that all conversations with her boys are at a laconic, instrumental level. Interestingly, the subject she would most like to discuss deeply with them is the Holocaust. Ruth specifically expressed her attempts at building a world of "only good" for her sons.

The transgenerational transmission of Holocaust trauma is presumably playing a background role, intensifying her anxiety over her sons possibly dying in the army, motivating her to throw body and soul into creating a protective environment. Ruth is perhaps thus clearly voicing what other parents demonstrated through their descriptions.

Despite the Holocaust being mentioned in only three interviews, it is there at the core in the family and national background, nurtured by collective memory, its roots even reaching back to the Binding of Isaac.

To understand the unconscious defences at work under these conditions, I touch on several emotional dynamics as developed by Freud and Melanie Klein, through Ronald Fairbairn, to David Scharff and other theorists involved in the transgenerational transmission of trauma.

Freud (1915d, p. 150) explained that repression is not an event that takes place once but demands persistent expenditure of force, without which "the success of the repression would be jeopardized, so that a fresh act of repression would be necessary". He explains that harsh emotional charges from the past will join with, and activate, traumatic charges of similar emotional quality found in the psyche, including content unconsciously passed down from previous generations (Brenner, 2014; Kogan, 1995; Volkan, 2012; Volkan & Greer, 2002). The urge to return, in the present, occurs as resisting content from the past, even when that same content is no longer threatening (Freud, 1914).

Freud (1921) also explained that identification is the original form with which the emotion retains its libidinal attachment to the object. Its internalization is an alternative to this link. Melanie Klein (1946) identified what she termed "splitting": an unconscious emotional process occurring in the psyche, which cannot contain its parts perceived as "good" with those perceived as "bad". Through projective identification, internal objects and relationships experienced as too painful for the psyche are attributed to another. In Klein's view, these relationships typify all early relationships in the individual.

Bion (1967) expanded understanding of projective identification and internalization, explaining that the individual who has processed these parts inside her/himself, identifies with them and becomes their container. An example is parents who internalize a child's extreme anxiety, contain it, "digest" it, and return it to the child in a less threatening or enduring form. According to Fairbairn (1944), Ogden (1989, 1994), and Scharff and Scharff (2014), this projection may be to achieve additional objectives, such as communication or better coping with pain caused by the content, and to store them in a place safe from internalized destructive drives.

As detailed in chapter four, psychoanalysis has identified these mechanisms in couple and family relationships (Dicks, 1967; Scharff & Scharff, 2014), explaining through them how traumatic emotional material is transferred to the next generation (Faimberg, 2005; Gampel, 2005; Scharff & Scharff, 2014).

The transgenerational transference of Holocaust trauma

This theoretical infrastructure provides a basis for understanding how the Holocaust wends its way into the conscious and unconscious emotional world and impacts emotional relationships and behaviours transgenerationally.

In states of extreme trauma, the emotional worlds aroused are so extreme that the psyche is unable to absorb and contain them. Instead, it is forced to split and project them outwards (Klein, 1946). However, as these are "parts of the self", they do not disappear but must be deposited in another individual.

Depositing overwhelming experiences in children's infantile psyches means that the children accept what the parents have projected onto them and adopt these unprocessed emotions as though they are their own. They remain unconscious of the fact that the distress, anxiety, and forceful mourning they may sense at times are not actually entirely their own and do not derive from a current situation, but are aggravated as a result of the projected emotional world of the first generation (Brenner, 2014; Faimberg, 2005; Kogan, 1995; Mann-Shalvi, 2007a, 2007b; Volkan, 2012; Volkan & Greer, 2002).

Transgenerational transmission was mentioned by Anna Freud and Dorothy Burlingham (1942) in breakthrough research into the unconscious influences passed from mothers to their children during the Blitz in London in World War II. Sullivan (1953) deepened understanding of how maternal anxiety becomes the child's anxiety.

Volkan explains that trauma shared by a large group, under conditions where an enemy intentionally causes its victims pain, shame, humiliation and helplessness, may create specific unidentified processes in the identity of the offspring of survivors of the group, causing them unconsciously to execute tasks without their consciousness (Volkan & Greer, 2002, p. 10).

Auerhahn and Laub (1998) explained that a massive trauma such as the Holocaust is engraved at the psychotic level—that is, without an associative organization typical of normal memories. Thus, the trauma passes from generation to generation, continuing to torture the psyches of the offspring, wordlessly and without the possibility of representation. The force of the horror cannot be perceived, digested, or contained and is therefore transmitted down the generations in its raw form, waiting for emotional processing.

Faimberg (2005) called the process of transgenerational trauma "the telescoping of generations". According to Freud, in order to experience separateness from the other an individual must have a well-balanced narcissistic psyche—that is, a regulated self-love, which occurs in the encounter between the pleasure principle and the reality principle. If this emotional regulation does not take place and object relations are based on self-love, the individual adopts, for her or his ego, that aspect of the external object which causes pleasure or provides needs and drives. Those that cause unpleasure will tend to be hated and will relate to that aspect in the other as "non-ego". In other words, in love relationships based on this dynamic, the other is loved for representing aspects of the subject's self. In such cases, there is no sense of space between ego and object, which allows the individual to begin accepting loss.

This mechanism operates in transgenerational transmission of extreme trauma, such as the Holocaust. In such a case, the parents often identify with everything good in the child and take possession of its positive identity. However, those parts or experiences they find impossible to contain and process in any way are not acknowledged; they project everything they experience as bad within themselves into the child and relate it to the child's negative identity. The child, then, becomes hated not only for being the other or different but, paradoxically, because the child's history is in congruence with their own hated history and everything they could not accept as their own in the process of narcissistic regulation. The child is then left with no space to develop its own individual identity.

Unconsciously, the trauma and its outcomes seem to "invade" the second, and often even the third, generation's psyche. According to Faimberg (2005), transgenerational transference empties the psyche of the second generation from its emotional world and its authentic identification of its needs, feelings, and wishes and invades that generation as though the trauma were actually experienced first-hand by it. Since this is an unconscious process, the second and even third generation can only sense the transgenerational transference through experiences of emptiness, loss of their way, automatic functioning, purposelessness, the sense of pleasing others, etc.[3]

This is one of many ways in which past and present intertwine and are unconsciously transmitted to the second and third generation. Survivors' offspring find themselves living the emotional lives of the previous generation, but in the current reality (Kogan, 1995). Thus, states exist in which emotional force attributed to events occurring in the present can draw on, and be intensified by, the chain of traumatic events that occurred in the past, transmitted unconsciously between generations and "magnetized" onto a current event (Brenner, 2014; Faimberg, 2005; Kogan, 1995; Laub, 1998; Laub & Lee, 2003; Mann-Shalvi, 2007a, 2007b).

As this is an unconscious process, it is not surprising that there was no conscious mention of the Holocaust by parents in relation to their extreme anxiety, helplessness, and guilt over a son's possible future death. This insight may give rise to resistance from an unconscious reaction to approaching the difficult content. For instance, we might expect that the impact on subsequent generations would exist only among families of actual Holocaust survivors. What is apparent, though, is that not only is the Holocaust engraved on the hearts of survivors and their offspring, but the trauma of it continues to live on in the hearts of anyone growing up in Israel, exposed to the Israeli-Jewish heritage, to events occurring in Israel, and therefore to the emotional intensity that is so hard for the psyche to contain (Ben-Ari & Levy-Schreiber, 2000; Guvrin, 1935; Segev, 1991; Shapira, 1997). Much has been written on this subject, some of it echoing the emotional baggage found in remarks made by interviewed parents relative to their sons' future recruitment.

For example, Anita Shapira (1997) claims that the population of the newly established country of Israel showed ambivalence towards Holocaust survivors—those who had just returned from the inferno yet represented the foreign. Warily, it could be said that Israelis have fallen in love with the image of the victim and adopted it, while simultaneously rejecting it and renouncing "the old Jews".

Numerous films present the female Holocaust survivor as mentally ill and unable to function other than as a mother in the limited space of her home, and even unable to fully fill that role (Steir-Livny, 2011). The female survivor is often presented as "a dominant, silencing, castrating mother who makes her children's lives miserable . . . an image that continues . . . to this very day" (p. 509). An attitude of disgust and rejection are also shown towards helplessness in male Jews—a helplessness that connects with stereotypical negative traits of the Diaspora Jew as passive and wimpy (Shapira, 1997).

Steir-Livny (2011) described how the horrors of the Holocaust initially constituted a source of loathing and repudiation. Towards the close of the 1940s, the phenomenon of forced prostitution of Jewish women in the Holocaust embodied the height of humiliation and Nazi regime perversion, adding the dimension of sexual stimulus. This perception surfaced in the public discourse despite being a marginal phenomenon in the Holocaust reality.

There may possibly be an affinity between this content and the "solution" found by mothers in my study, with their patterns of dominant maternal overprotectiveness, over-pampering, and castration of the masculine individuation process. Could this be additional testimony to the unconscious expression of Holocaust trauma content in Israeli motherhood when the latter encounters the emotional content of a threat to life? If there is truth to this insight, then we need to understand what allows Holocaust content to be revived with such agitation in current life, and how this content connects with the issue of recruitment.

In the 1980s, through the media, the Holocaust ceased being an event distant from the past and became a presence in the everyday collective memory. First-person testimonies of Holocaust survivors began to be published, as well as second-generation narratives describing the impact on their own lives. And in 2014, Israel's minister of education, Shai Piron, decided to introduce a Holocaust study programme, from nursery-school age up. Could we be witnessing the return of the repressed? As Freud explained:

> The vanished affect comes back in its transformed shape as social anxiety, moral anxiety and unlimited self-reproaches; the rejected idea is replaced by a substitute by displacement, often a displacement on to something very small or indifferent. . . . [1915d, p. 156]

Guilt feelings are indeed one of the central emotions that Holocaust survivors and their offspring must cope with: survivors may blame themselves and express shame for not doing enough to save their relatives, or accept responsibility for group shame as Jews who did not oppose the Nazis.

Primo Levi, who survived Auschwitz, wrote how, when it was all over, they started to acknowledge the fact that they had done nothing or had taken insufficient action against the system in which they had chanced: "Consciously or not, he [the survivor] feels accused and judged, compelled to justify and defend himself" (Levi, 1963).

The motif of Jews as lambs to the slaughter,[4] to death in gas chambers, was cemented during Israel's early decades as a fundamental image of exterminated Jews. In parallel, a blaming finger was pointed at those who survived, as though they must have done something immoral. These complex perceptions and modes of representation of Holocaust victims and survivors remain as part of the scars comprising the national emotional makeup (Guvrin, 1935; Shapira, 1997; Steir-Livny, 2011).

Most of Israel's citizens were united by the Holocaust trauma through consciousness of a shared destiny and mutual responsibility. "In our generation's consciousness", notes Schweid (1990), "the Holocaust of eastern European Jewry and the establishment of the State of Israel are linked, and some even tend to see them as cause and effect." Carol Gilligan (personal communication, 2001) emphasized the need "to understand the importance of the Israeli soldier protecting his family, against the background of the Jewish father from the Holocaust who did not succeed in protecting his family".

Holocaust and resurrection

The ideological Zionist narrative creates a vital affinity between the Holocaust and Israel's establishment and robustness. Appropriately, the Israeli identity is interpreted as one aimed at overcoming such events. The historian Tom Segev (1991) details numerous examples where the Holocaust's memory is harnessed for political needs, as well as its impact on social processes, military procedures, and political approaches in the international arena. This is also shown in the affinity between the IDF and the Holocaust experience as it penetrates the personal narratives of Holocaust survivors.

Naftali Lau-Lavie was a child in the extermination camps. He saved his five-year-old brother and emigrated to Israel during the struggle for Israel's independence. He worked as a journalist and then as an attaché and spokesman for Ministers of Defence Moshe Dayan and Lapid Peres; he became a diplomat and participated in the peace negotiations with Egypt; and he headed the World Jewish Restitution Organization handling the return of Jewish property to Holocaust survivors. In his book *The Nation as a Lion* (Lau-Lavie, 1993), Naftali relates his life story and allows a close encounter with how the experience of helplessness from the narrative of the Binding of Isaac, perpetuated in the Holocaust, was countered through immigrating to Israel, with its military force.

In a chilling account, Naftali describes the moment of separation from his father, the last Chief Rabbi of Piotrekov, Poland, who chose to stay with the members of his community on the journey to the concentration camps instead of trying to flee with his own family:

> On coming home, I found father sitting in his study, a small book open before him. . . To me he seemed more lost in thought than in the book's content. Finally he sighed and said, "That's it." We looked at each other for several seconds without exchanging a word, until I sank into the deep armchair next to him and burst into tears. . . . Father did not try to calm me, but turned to me as the firstborn son of the household.

Naftali's father related to him as a mature, responsible youngster. Together, they looked straight in the "eye" of the looming "binding":

> It was the first time for many months that my father came over to me and kissed me on the forehead. . . . A warm tear fell from his eye and landed on my cheek. "We will behave the way our forefather Jacob did when he readied his family for the anticipated encounter with his hostile brother, Esau." Jacob divided the family into three camps, hoping that at least one would remain intact . . .

Naftali describes that night's Sabbath[5] evening meal, with his mother and his brothers, and the last words he remembers through the confusion and emotion flooding him:

> The two of us stood alone, facing each other. I was a lad of sixteen, setting out alone on a life journey that could be very short, and at most I would have to fight for my place in the world. Before me stood father, a man of fifty, a public leader, with rich life experience.

Stocked with the love of a father who believed in his ability, belief in the Supreme Godly father watching over him, and a sense of meaning and belonging with a history of thousands of years, along with clear instructions on which way he should be going, Naftali succeeds in fulfilling his father's wishes. He managed to save himself and his younger brother, who eventually became Israel's Chief Rabbi.

The events he experienced in the Holocaust are clearly inseparable from his experiences as an Israeli soldier. Among other incidents, he talks of how, in April 1974, he found himself in the coastal town of Maalot in northern Israel as terrorists took control of the local school and murdered an infant boy and his parents as well as another twenty-one school children, injuring seventy others. Naftali describes the thoughts passing through his mind as negotiations to release the hostages took place with the terrorists:

> When the firing stopped, I ran after Moshe Dayan to the building. Tens of boys and girls and several adults lay dead or injured on the floor, and several sat leaning against the wall screaming for help. The horrific scene sent me back thirty years, to scenes I hadn't found release from ever since Auschwitz and Buchenwald. I stood there, helpless, feeling my legs collapsing beneath me. I hurried outside and sat on a curbstone. . . . A soldier held out his water canteen and I took a few sips until I felt I could stand steadily again.

The Israeli warrior, who can protect his own life and that of his family, is pitched against Naftali's father or grandfather, who couldn't do a thing. Unlike during the Holocaust, the Israeli soldier is an answer to the helplessness of the schoolchildren and of Naftali, who once again faces the horrors of the Holocaust. When Naftali read my interpretation of his emotions, he admitted wholeheartedly that I had hit the nail on the head.

This next description comes from an article in a daily newspaper, by Felix Frisch and the AP Agency. It relates to the memorial flyover conducted by the Israel Air Force above Auschwitz,[6] demonstrating more than all else how past, present, and future merge for the Jewish people in general, and Israelis in particular.

> . . . the flyover was led by Brigadier General Amir Eshel whose family was murdered in Poland, and as his plane flew over Auschwitz, the words he spoke rang out through loudspeakers across the extermination camp:
>
> > "We, pilots of the Israel Air Force, flying in the skies above the camp of horrors, arose from the ashes of the millions of victims and shoulder their silent cries, salute their courage, and promise to be the shield of the Jewish people and its nation, Israel." [*Yediot Aharonot*, 5 September 2003]

As the jets flew over the camp, the names of the Jews brought to the camp on 4 September 1943 were read out.

Ten years later, the pilots met and described how the flyover impacted each of them. Their words merged inseparably the Holocaust and the current Israeli reality. Brigadier General Eshel had this to say to the delegation:

> That moment, when we successfully demonstrated the narrative of the Jewish people, is etched and tangible even today. As the progeny of an ancient, complex nation, which numerous times has been

> on the brink of annihilation, we roused questions and thoughts on Israeli identity, on our resilience and vitality, unparalleled throughout human history. The photograph . . . has taken hold in our consciousness, and expresses the uniquely Israeli composition that mingles sorrow and grandeur, pain and pride, and creates hope. The Israel Air Force is the clearest of all manifestations of this nation's path: from the dreadful nullification to unprecedented power. We, members of the air force, are privileged to bear responsibility and infuse the spirit that turns hopes and wishes into true ability that ensures life . . . the significance of the flyover has penetrated the national consciousness in Israel and in Jewish communities overseas.
>
> I look at that photograph every day. It is a kind of compass, the balance scales, the important versus the irrelevant, a charging power that requires no words or explanations. I look at it, and know we will overcome.[7]

From the psychoanalytic angle, an action such as the flyover can be related to as a form of enactment (Laplanche & Pontalis, 1973)—a concrete manifestation that takes the place of a symbolic expression that, as Freud explained, replaces the instinctive reaction for revenge. The action derives from the internal arena's periphery of wishes and phantasies and allows relieving them in the present, with a sense of urgency amplified by the refusal to acknowledge their recurring source and nature.

These examples serve as a tip of an iceberg and demonstrate the multidimensionality of the connection between the Holocaust, the IDF, and the State of Israel at the personal and public levels. They also clarify my theory that this emotional burden also seeps into unconscious levels of Israeli parenting.

It is important to emphasize that the Holocaust survivors themselves provide widely diverse interpretations of the harsh experiences they endured, and they reach completely different life-lesson conclusions. Their relationship to the personal and national connection between Holocaust and the military is accordingly derived.

Holocaust memory in Israel

The way the Holocaust is memorialized and perpetuated in Israel through media, education, and culture creates significant impact on both children and parents and is worthy of review.

In an interview in 2014,[8] Saul Friedlander, a historian and researcher of the Holocaust and Third Reich (Friedlander, 1983), dissociated himself from the way Holocaust memory is currently handled in Israel. Friedlander experienced the Holocaust as a child in a Catholic monastery. He denounces what he calls political manipulations of the Holocaust—trips to Auschwitz and "demonstrations of flyovers and ceremonies", which, for him, cheapen tragic pain without processing it.

Zuckerman (2001) pointed to the gap between the attitudes towards victimization of Holocaust survivors as a topic, and attitudes towards the distress felt by the individual survivor:

> Since the Zionist ideology relies on total immersion to negate the Diaspora connection, the Holocaust victim . . . must be absorbed into the Zionist ideology through negation . . . Regarding the perished, this demand could no longer be made: they quickly became an immense mass of anonymous objects ("the six million") and the object of ideological accusatory piety ("If only the State of Israel had readied itself on time").

Zuckerman describes how the survivors filled this national "requirement" by behaving during the day like Israelis, but returning at night to their recurring nightmares. This corresponds to the understanding that traumatic emotional baggage was suppressed at both the personal and national levels.

Yehuda Elkana,[9] who also survived Auschwitz, identifies the existence of existential anxiety rooted in the Holocaust as fundamental to attitudes towards the Palestinians. This existential anxiety is projected onto the Palestinians and reconstructed relative to them. He says:

> Lately I am increasingly convinced that . . . the socio-political factor driving Israeli society's attitude towards the Palestinians [is] a *deep existential anxiety nurtured by a particular interpretation of the lessons of the Holocaust, and from the willingness to believe that the entire world is against us and we are the eternal victim* [emphasis added]. . . . From Auschwitz there came, symbolically speaking, two nations: a minority that claimed "*This* will never happen again" and a frightened, anxious majority that claimed "This will never happen *to us* again". [*Ha'aretz*,13 October 2012]

In 2014, two articles[10] appeared in a national daily newspaper, *Ha'aretz*, in which offspring of Holocaust survivors—Leah Eini and Yitzhak Schwartz—describe their childhoods under the pall of abusive Holocaust survivor parents. Both generalized, saying they are not just telling their personal stories but the story of "a generation with crazy parents, Holocaust survivors". In reaction, Holocaust researcher Leah

Steir-Livny[11] warned that the freedom to speak from personal experience in the name of a generational group can create a warped, erroneous memory of the entire group. She referred to herself as the granddaughter of a Lodz Ghetto survivor, a gentle soul who devoted large parts of his life to assisting others, a trait shared by his friends.

The psychoanalyst Viviane Chetrit-Vatine (2014) writes of treating survivors and the later generations:

> Humanity after the Shoah[12] . . . is wounded by the events that have traversed it and continue to traverse it. The closely knit structures of the family interwoven with the social structures are being transformed. . . . The organizing myths of reference are no longer so obviously adequate. The analyses that we conduct are intended for people . . . who are profoundly discontent and sometimes struggling to survive at all.

Even though the Holocaust experience is continually perpetuated through memorial events and books, it is evident that it is still insufficiently emotionally processed. French historian Pierre Nora (1993) wrote: "We speak so much of memory, because so little is left of it." The greater the inflation in formal memorial sites, the more the spontaneous authentic memory will diminish.

In his response to Heidegger's paper about the problem of Jewish "representation", philosopher Jean-François Lyotard (1988) explains that a person may be able to forget the crime precisely through its "representation". In this way, the representation of Auschwitz through words and images is a way of forgetting it. This can be seen, for example, in the accounts of young children about the war era collected by the Central Historical Committee for the purpose of understanding the situation more fully, while allowing children the freedom that would release them from the burden of memory (Alshatien, 2014). The emotional worlds of the children revealed in their stories are far more meaningful than the big picture, presenting a different documentation from the motives recurring in Israeli education systems. A similar approach is taken by Claude Lanzmann in his movie, *Shoah,* with its rejection of representation. In fact, almost all the testimonies indicate the impossibility of representing the destruction, where each representation is to some extent a symptom of oblivion.

The horrors of the Holocaust are naturally the focus of all attention, but at the 74th Congress of French-speaking Psychoanalysts (Montreal, 2014), Robert Asseo and Sylvie Dreyfus-Asseop discussed the impact of laws directed against Jews in France between 1940 to 1942, even before the implementation of "The final solution". According to them, the effect on Jews—but not only on Jews—of the cumulative trauma of a series of orders damaging the rights of Jews was desubjectivation, an action that attacks individuals' subjectivation, alienating them from society and also from themselves. I think survivors experienced situations so much more traumatic that they overrode the marginalization and distancing that cause desubjectivation. Nonetheless, such a dynamic may continue to be activated in their psyches and transmitted unconsciously to the coming generations.[13]

The same content that fell into the abyss of oblivion continues to echo in the hearts of the survivors' children and grandchildren, seeking expression in current content that will make this possible without consciousness of its source. One avenue for this is in parenting sons in Israel.

Further thoughts

The publicized number of fallen in Israel's battles and hostilities is over 23,000. When asked when that count starts, most people would probably respond with "1948", that being the establishment of Israel. Surprise and shock greet the information that the count starts from 1860,[14] a fact concealed on Memorial Days. The impression is that this is the number killed in wars and hostilities, which creates an intensified experience of helplessness, loss anxiety, and mourning. It is a reality that supports the understanding that parental emotional intensity relative to recruitment of sons does not arise from the current reality but is aggravated by transmission of unprocessed traumatic content from the past.

Again, the number of dead in traffic accidents in Israel is four times higher than the fallen in all the wars and hostilities Israel has experienced, yet the parents interviewed hardly mentioned being anxious about their sons' lives as a result of their driving in the future.

It is important to note that feeling anxious is natural when a child, barely more than an adolescent, leaves home; it is even more so when a son leaves for commando service, which includes using weapons and the possibility of taking part in military actions. It is reasonable to assume that if parents' anxiety remained tied to the actual numbers of fallen and injured from the time of Israel's establishment, and took into account that in the army the sons learn defence skills and protective measures when using the most advanced weapons, parents could contain their anxiety. It would then be reasonable to assume that we would come across varying levels of anxiety, based on Israel's security situation at the time of the interview, and that the strength of parents' anxiety would rise as the recruitment date drew closer.

But, as noted, we found a different picture, one that makes it important to try to understand what could activate the transgenerational conscious and unconscious baggage linked to the Holocaust in the psyches of parents of sons, intensifying their anxiety to an extent that it accompanies parenthood and couplehood from the moment of learning that the fetus is male.

Perhaps it is precisely because the IDF's strength is associated with the need prevent a repeat of the Holocaust that recruitment draws unprocessed anxiety from the past from the depths of the parents' psyches. Parents flooded with anxiety are unaware that it is sourced in the Holocaust, among other things; they attribute their emotions to the possibility of life-threatening risk to their sons via future recruitment.

Additionally, the generation born in the early twentieth century, who helplessly experienced the Holocaust first-hand, conveyed to their children clear messages about the need to be warrior males when needed—yet they conveyed this need as deriving from anxiety over a repeat of the Holocaust. As surfaces from the interviews, in their youth fathers had strongly identified with this message and therefore served in fighting units. But as fathers, they find themselves in conflict because of the incompatibility between their identity as consolidated and their current parenthood—a conflict that makes it harder for them to identify unequivocally with the traditional role of the warrior male who similarly educates his sons.

The difficulty in conveying a clear message, as already detailed, allows unprocessed anxiety from the past to surface in its "current guise". Thus, the parents project onto their sons deep feelings of helpless victimhood relative to the danger of destruction, weighing the sons' shoulders down with unconscious and unprocessed forceful anxieties transmitted from earlier generations but wrapped in current content.

These understandings raise a question: what are the unconscious emotional processes of a young man receiving such powerful emotional messages in conflictual forms? What impact do these processes have? The issue of the path taken by the young Israeli male, in light of these powerful complex messages, from the time of maturity and all the way through to his combat service, is even more sharply focused on in Part II.

Notes

1. In Israel, where extreme descriptions of incidents in concentration camps abound, a localized slang developed that refers to individuals directly affected by the Holocaust but without the extreme experiences as "light Holocaust survivor". The phrase expresses numerous unspoken and sometimes unconscious emotions, such as guilt, or is a means of creating dissociation to avoid encountering the emotional baggage surrounding speakers admitting that their parents are Holocaust survivors in the fullest sense.

2. *Tzabar*: Hebrew for prickly pear—a nickname given to Israeli-born individuals, describing a stereotypical "prickly on the outside" (i.e., tough, resilient) "but soft on the inside" characterization.

3. In fact, Faimberg's explanation parallels that offered in earlier chapters on the essence of the projective identification process. The difference between them is that the first is based on the Freudian understanding of the dynamic, the second on relational understanding of the dynamic.

4. "Going like lambs to their slaughter" is a concept from Isaiah 53: 7 [sheep to the slaughter] adapted by Abba Kovner in December 1941 in a circular calling members of the Vilna Ghetto not to go to their deaths "like lambs to the slaughter". These words now express national trauma (Segev, 1991).

5. Friday evening: the Jewish Sabbath begins at sundown on Friday, ending after sunset on Saturday.

6. YouTube: "Israel Flyover Over Auschwitz" [with English subtitles]: https: // www.youtube.com/watch?v=lfv3jsLGzL0

7. From the official IDF website: www.idf.il/1133-19563-he/Dover.aspx

8. The "Crossing Israel" TV programme with Kobi Meidan, Channel 23, shown on 22 and 25 May 2014.

9. Yehuda Elkana is an outspoken critic of Israeli educational methods for sciences and of Holocaust education and memorialization in Israel.

10. "Craving Life and Revenge, They Ruined Our Childhood", *Ha'aretz* magazine, 23 May 2014; "Coming Out", *Ha'aretz* magazine, 6 June 2014.

11. *Ha'aretz* magazine, 13 June 2014.

12. *Shoah*: "annihilation", or more commonly, "Holocaust".

13. Thanks to Dr Michel Granek for reporting from the conference and formulating this summary.

14. This is a puzzling date. Perhaps it expresses the wish to create a temporal, continuous ideological narrative from the days when Jewish towns and villages began expanding in Palestine in the late nineteenth century, and the resulting hostilities and attacks by Arabs, through to the modern wars Israel has fought. This outlines a much longer line of Jewish sovereignty than that from formal statehood in 1948.

PART II

VICISSITUDES OF A MAN'S LIFE

CHAPTER SIX

Lack of maturity versus hunger for maturity

In Part I, we saw that the Israeli reality—that young male adolescents are recruited by law into military combat service—creates an emotional trap for parents: if they fulfil their parental task and raise a son with high levels of physical, cognitive, and emotional capability and a masculine identity separate from theirs, they will themselves have contributed a great deal to their son's recruitment to combat service, which could put his life at stake.

The unconscious conflict finds its solution unconsciously as the splitting of contradictory parental tasks shifts from an intrapsychic conflict to an interpersonal one between them, burdening the couple relationship with tension. The maternal pattern of overprotectiveness creates the illusion of an ideal world for their sons, which sabotages the consolidation of a separate identity. In parallel, fathers become mute and even concealed. Added to all this is a tension that typifies the couple relationship relative to the issue of their sons.

Several powerful processes of intergenerational trauma were also observed, related to Jewish and Israeli history, which populate, at the conscious and unconscious levels, the psyches of parents of sons.

The dynamic understandings can be summarized as follows:

1. By splitting the intrapsychic conflict between opposing parental tasks and turning that conflict interpersonal between the couple, *each parent experiences individual relief* but the couple relationship is burdened with continuous tension.
2. The conflictual parenting patterns between the parents keep the son from adopting the masculine combat identity while growing up and until recruitment, thus creating the illusion of control and

distance from combat service content, which *allows the parents to pacify their loss anxiety and current experience of parental helplessness, as well as anxieties that draw on, and are intensified by, intergenerational transmission of Holocaust trauma.*

3. Simultaneously, this parental dynamic *can result in the experience of developmental deficiency and a longing for a macho-heroic identity, causing the son's attraction to that combat identity; on recruitment, the son will adopt it unswervingly and serve in a combat unit.*
4. The division of roles between parents *allows the son to internalize, from the parents as one parental unit, those messages he needs for his maturity* but sets them into a rigid system of roles, in repetitive emotional patterns and relationships.

It is also important to remember that in the interviews some parents voiced the experienced conflict accompanying their behaviour towards their sons, such as those fathers who felt resistance caused by the mothers' behaviour, or mothers who expressed their feeling of discomfort over their own behaviour. For example, Hedy described how she raises them to not conform to the necessary masculine military profile, but then conflict surfaces in her: "I wasn't raised that way."

The following chapters deal with the Israeli soldier—his transition from a protective home, through military service, to re-entry into civilian life, where he must function as a mature Israeli man.[1] This is not a comprehensive picture but merely the start of a discourse, and it gives non-Israeli readers a view of Israeli reality that is not shown in the media.

The impact of parenting on structuring a son's identity

Psychoanalytic theory offers a means to understand how the parenting patterns shown in the interviews can impact the son's development, personality, and functionality.

It is important to emphasize that the terms "maternal" and "paternal" also relate to the fatherly aspect in mothers and the mothering aspect in fathers. Moreover, when the father "takes on the role of mother", the mother finds herself adopting the paternal role. This is consistent with the understanding that the emotional intrapsychic trap in which Israeli parents of sons find themselves thrusts them into turning this into an intersubjective conflict in their couple relationship and that sometimes they exchange roles.

In terms of the unconscious dynamic, this is a dual oedipal conflict, this time from the parents' perspective. Ogden (1989) explained that as part of the developmental resolution of the parents' oedipal conflict, in each parent is an internalized image of the other parent. Thus, when the mother becomes an object of passion, the image of the father who sets boundaries and prohibitions is also internalized, and vice versa. In accordance with the dominant paternal and maternal aspect in each parent, and with the bisexuality inherent in each of us and its position on the scale, the balance will determine the choice of object in each boy or girl.

Psychoanalytic theory (e.g., Fairbairn, 1944, 1963; Freud, 1895; Klein, 1937a, 1937b; Winnicott, 1960, 1968) places great emphasis on the experiences of the infant's earliest years—first and foremost on the infant's relationship with its mother and father, or the adults in the infant's immediate sphere of contact. Through these primary relationships the infant begins to experience deeper feelings of love, trust, hate, envy, fear, and suspicion. These early experiences of relationship, alongside inherited components, have a great impact on consolidating behaviour as adults and beliefs concerning the self and others. Early experiences also affect the personal relationships adults will be able to build, as well as how well they may realize inherited capabilities and psychological potential, the fulfilment of which depends largely on an individual's sense of gratification and self-esteem. These early experiences are the basis of the development of individuals' internal perceptions of self and their understanding of other people and of the world in which they live. These experiences are also the basis of the individual's instinctive feelings of excitement, tension, gratification, and pleasure, as well as unavoidable frustration and suffering.

Independent, gratified mature identity becomes possible when there is a balance between aspects of the personality that emphasize its individuation—a "doing" emotional attitude—and those that emphasize its fusion with the other—a "being" emotional attitude. A state of balance between the two allows the development of complex emotional skills and optimal states of mature independence. The process of separation by the son from the mother, and growing closeness to the father, is of primary importance in achieving balance in these processes (Erlich, 1990, 1998).

Fairbairn (1952) understood that, because of the basic need for relationships, an individual's psyche organizes itself throughout life on the basis of the many facets of the parents internalized by the individual while he or she was growing up. The external object relations become internal object relations. Parents' authenticity and the complex discourse with them thus allow development of multiple facets that potentially exist within the child's personality and the ability for internal discourse leading to creativity and manifestations of the unique self in the child.

Proper development requires from the outset the presence of a mother's active adjustment to her infant, responding to its emotional and physical needs through uncomplaining dedication. Over time, the mother must adjust herself to the infant's requirements, according to the infant's growing ability to cope with frustration when it feels those needs are not being met (Winnicott, 1969, 1971).

Frustration that matches the infant's, and later the child's, stage of development causes the child to seek alternative solutions not provided by the mother, allowing the development of creativity, capabilities, and ability to understand external reality and test one's strengths, all of which promote children's development and familiarization with their own unique individuality.

The early infantile experiences include coexistence between perspectives of the mother as an environment and as an object. In infancy, however, the first perspective is one in which the infant's experience of the mother as part of the self is dominant. As development progresses, the relationship between these perspectives changes (Winnicott, 1968). In fact, the fusion states of mind between infant and mother occurs only in phantasy. In the dialectic process, reality enters into the relationship, and a space is created between reality and phantasy where subjectivity, personal meaning, symbols, and imagination develop and can exist (Winnicott, 1962).

The infant seeking a relationship with the mother—or primary caregiver—will inevitably encounter disappointment, as when the mother cannot be constantly available to gratify needs. A mother who responds without too much seduction and can set boundaries without being too hostile and rejecting, strengthens the infant's self with feelings of confidence, abundance, love, calm, and gratification (Scharff & Scharff, 2014). A mother who nurtures too much, holds back in anxiety, gives too much attention, or floods with inappropriate luring is an exciting mother who floods the infant; the infant then feels anxiety, dependence, and longing for relief. A mother who is depressive, too tired, and angry when she must react to her infant leads to an infant who feels rejected, angry, and abandoned.

A pattern embedded in the early life stages is translated in more complex ways in adult life. The child's need for independence changes over time and requires parallel parental adaptation. These understandings raise tough questions about the impact of emotional messages emitted by parents when they prevent their sons from experiencing these processes.

In the interviews, a focal motif was "pampering" sons and a maternal desire to create a world in which sons would always be happy. This might have several consequences.[2]

When raised in a world "where all is good", a son may not develop sufficient consciousness of his limitations and drawbacks, with a sense of being perfect and that the world needs to adapt itself to him. "Spoilt sons" is the term used by Lieblich (2001) for "light" outcomes; "narcissistic" is the psychoanalytic term for more extreme outcomes.

Erlich (1998, p. 141) explains that narcissists cannot bear their sense of imperfection and their limitations, and therefore position themselves as if they need no one. They create a bubble around themselves containing all they need, and everything is experienced as good and appropriately reflects whichever aspects in themselves they admire. The greater these traits in narcissists, the less they perceive themselves as being dependent. The myth of self-gratification negates object relations and the ability to perceive the real absence needed for symbolization, claims Erlich. This description parallels that of mothers detailing a world in which their sons do not encounter need, frustration, or inability while the fathers' presence represents order, law, and the absent boundary.

Lewow (2011) explains that unconditional love may be far from benign. It is love that does not allow seeing what is harmful, painful, or negative in the loved one, simultaneously preserving the sense of belonging to, and caring for, that loved one. According to Lewow, such love, on the part of parents, educators, and therapists, constitutes an important factor in causing the psychic stress and behavioural disorders from which these children suffer. By incorrectly using the concept of "understanding", parents back up their children's severe violent behaviour in school, instead casting blame on others—if only so their children avoid bearing the outcome of their actions. Parents conduct logical and emotional acrobatics just to escape feeling pain and anxiety over their sons' behaviour. In such cases, the term "good" becomes distorted and, instead of an experience of cohesion and growth, it turns into a feeling of pleasant comfort and relief, as expressed by the interviewed parents. Parallel to this, and extremely damaging in its impact, an experience containing difficulty is identified by these parents as "a bad experience".

Psychic well-being requires encountering the parents' subjectivity, along with all its emotions, thoughts, wishes, and abilities. Such encounters allow the developing child to understand emotions and internalize a stance of "you know what I feel, even when I want or feel the opposite of what you want or feel". Such internalization allows sharing emotions with the other without fearing that "my feelings are your feelings" (Lewow, 2011, pp. 21–22).

Love that does not avoid conflictual states and allows expressing criticism or setting boundaries enables children to identify otherness, which, in turn, allows mutual understanding between them and their parents and the ability to negotiate different stances and find alternatives. Without separateness between parents and children, relationships are created in which there is room for only one type of emotion—when, for example, one gives and the other receives, or one acknowledges and the other receives acknowledgment—and otherness is enabled only through role exchange (Benjamin, 1995).

Proper development requires an increasing ability to acknowledge otherness. To form mature relationships in which there is room for both the parents' and the son's true selves, it is necessary to create a relational space that allows the personal uniqueness of mother, father, and son to encounter each other and the space shared by them.

There are critical periods when this psychic organization comes about; one of these is around the age of three to five years, when the Oedipus complex is experienced. The boy's great love at the outset of his life is his mother, and in order to keep her entirely his, and out of envy towards the father for his intimacy with her from which he is excluded, the son wishes to be rid of the father, killing him in childhood phantasy (Laplanche & Pontalis, 1973, p. 282). Fearing the father will take revenge by castrating him, as he imagines must have happened to his sister, he transfers his identity from mother to father—making this stage significant in the son's process of adopting a masculine identity. For the process to occur, both parents must, of course, enable and support it. The oedipal stage fills a basic need in structuring personality, especially when building the superego responsible for judgement and censorship, norms and values. The ego-ideal is responsible for integrating narcissism—the ideal self—and identification with parents as a model to which the self can try to adjust, conditions vital for the ability to understand human desires and wishes.

Internalized within the psyche of each parents is the figure of the other parent (Ogden, 1989), so the transition between the son's love of and identification with the mother and that with the father is not so acute. Even in the early stage of his great love for the mother, then, the son encounters within her that aspect of father internalized within her. This encounter paves the way for the son's identification with the father as an external object and its later internalization as part of shaping the son's masculine self.

During adolescence, sexual development arouses latent childhood sexuality, reopening the son's psyche to the oedipal dynamic; this time it is resolved through finding an alternative partner, instead of the mother, with whom to structure his own new family[3] (Kohlberg & Gilligan, 1972).

The interviews showed a pattern of muteness on the fathers' part relative to sons, and it is important to understand its significance for the latter. The psychoanalytic literature has not expanded on the emotional influence of the absent father figure on children in general, and sons in particular, even though Freud (1912–13) stated that in his perception, the father holds a vital function in founding the son's sense of confidence. He understood the longing for and the mature relationship with the father as a defensive compromise directed at overcoming castration anxiety while resolving the oedipal conflict as the son shapes his masculine identity.

André Green explains that the father in this relationship is not a realistic father—rather, the "father" includes all the father figures of previous generations, together with their emotional world and values—as manifested in the Bible when an individual's name is given together with the names of numerous ancestral generations. Green explains that, unlike the relationship with the father, the relationship with the mother is, first and foremost, physical and is always a reality—the metaphorical dimension does not have the same importance (Meadow & Green, 2006).

It is interesting, therefore, to consider what the Israeli–Jewish father figure symbolizes, especially because throughout history it has wavered between two poles: one, the leader, strong and confident; the other, the weak figure who cannot defend his family. Perhaps this has a role in the admiration Israeli sons feel towards their commanders and masculine battle figures.

In situations where both parents are in states of unresolved emotional conflict between complex emotions and contradictory tasks, maternal dominancy and paternal avoidance must impede the son's unconscious emotional internalization and integration of maternal and paternal objects and thus affect his feminine and masculine characteristics. We can also assume that these parental patterns make it difficult to successfully resolve the separation–individuation process and the oedipal conflict, and as a result, when such sons enlist in the army, they may well have reached a more immature developmental stage than they might have had they been raised in a system that enables them to distance and consolidate their personal identity.

Israeli society is typified by a transition from collective combative values to democratic values of individualism (Shafir & Peled, 1998). It is natural to assume, too, that had the sons grown up under parenting patterns that encourage independence, unique identity consolidation, and personal development, the transition to the military framework that nurtures collective identity for the sake of all would be accompanied by the sense of disparity and conflict. It is logical that these feelings are intensified if sons are raised in parenting patterns that overtly and covertly keep them from finding their own independence and their ability to resist what does not suit them and from adopting those Israeli masculine characteristics that correspond to the traits of a combat soldier.

Sons must cope, on recruitment, with a monolithic environment that is aggressive, total, and demanding, preferably one that they should encounter following satisfactory separation–individuation. From this perspective, recruitment constitutes the first significant separation, and enlistment becomes a central experience in shaping sons' mature identities (Lomsky-Feder & Ben-Ari, 1999).

While separation at this age parallels that, for example, of teenagers leaving for university in many other countries, the unique element in the Israeli situation is that the exit from an overprotective framework to the totality of the military framework is accompanied by realistic anxiety aggravated by unconscious traumatic intergenerational content, with all its attendant consequences.

We should also remember that the fathers, even if silent, are nonetheless Israeli combat males who have served on military missions. Also, the more the teenager grows—even if parts of his maturation are inhibited—the more he is exposed to a reality that is very different from that drawn by his mother. Through the education system he is exposed to the concept of the combat male who rescues. He may well be confused by these conflicting messages and perhaps doubt the source of parental authority, its validity, and the extent to which it represents the truth. It may be the conflict that pushes him, even involuntarily, to consolidate his independent identity. This confusion, or his consciousness of the delay that his parents are causing in his development, can cause a longing for that very maturity which manifests specifically through his military service, as it is during that service that he acknowledges and develops the masculine combat parts of his self that he was prevented from acknowledging while growing up.

Can he, however, connect those parts in an integrative manner to the softer or more feminine parts that were encouraged while he was being raised? The following examples relate to the characteristics at two poles of the axis.

I spoke with three soldiers on leave who had been involved in an operation that required tight cooperation between various military corps. Although they had not trained specifically for this situation, all three noted the degree of seriousness, professionalism, responsibility, and restraint they encountered not only in themselves but also in their comrades in arms: "a sense of being able to rely on the soldiers around them, and on their commanders". Although still gripped by the atmosphere of war, they spoke quietly, without ranting—my impression was that, indeed, in their personalities the masculine and feminine parts manifested well. This seemed to be an example where "the unconscious parental resolution" had, in fact, successfully raised sons connected to both these facets of identity, despite the conflict through which they had been transmitted.

On the other hand, an echo of the difficulty in the integrative existence of the male and female parts can be found in two cases I encountered in my clinic.

> Elad, aged forty, divorced and the father of a child, came for therapy as part of his search for his unique masculine identity. Elad described how his mother had protected him from his father, who occasionally tried to make his voice heard by way of educating and guiding his son. Elad also described how he can't keep a job, can't seem to learn, and can't even progress in sports, even though, as a youth, he had been considered a promising sports talent. He blurred his experiences of frustration, anxiety, poor self-image, and pain through frequent use of soft drugs. For him, internalizing the voice that his father had tried to emphasize—"don't give up in the face of adversity, don't run away just because of frustration"—was very difficult. Over several years of psychoanalytic therapy he was able to set words to the feelings that shamed him. He had been pampered as a child and had taken advantage of his mother's

protectiveness, even when a second voice within him said this was wrong, that he did want to succeed alone, enjoy his athletic prowess, and express his own opinion on various issues. Towards the end of therapy he was able to connect within himself to the image of his father, adopt his father's voice as a guiding one that would allow him to live, and leave his mother's voice as one that would enable a respite rather than castrate his capabilities. In line with these changes, he has been employed at the same workplace for several years, while simultaneously becoming active in raising his son.

Yair, aged twenty-five, came for therapy after his release from military duty. He was confused and unsure what he wanted to do in life. He viewed therapy as an enabling space where he could acknowledge the diverse parts of his personality and, accordingly, consolidate his way forward. Severe anxiety attacks were preventing him from sleeping or functioning. Eventually he was able to describe how he had grown up in a very protective and pampering atmosphere, with his father very much in the shadows. Nevertheless, any step that meant realizing his individualism was accompanied by a sense of betraying his parents, and distancing from them raised the anxiety that was transmitted by them to him. Processing such content allowed Yair to find his own path. He chose a profession, registered for higher education, and met his future wife. On completing his studies, he found employment and began his professional life. But each time he faced a significant step in realizing his individuality, such as meaningful promotion at work or the decision to have a child, he experienced almost paralysing anxiety, which brought additional issues to the surface from that same emotional world.

One of the symptoms I encounter among many young men in my clinical practice is the difficulty in obeying rules and laws: "Boundaries are meant for breaking . . . boundaries and rules are just a recommendation."

A 2004 article in the internet monthly *Auto* noted that in any single hour of driving, the average Israeli driver breaks more traffic laws than drivers in most of Europe. The article identifies the state in which the Israeli driver "does not want" at the conscious level to uphold norms of commitment on the roads, and it raises a question that echoes the situations described above: "Is this the outcome of an inability to bear frustration, a state of not receiving exactly what I want the moment that I want it?"

The possibility that the son's reaction to parenting behaviours could be developmental deficiency or the inability to live an independent adult life is echoed in two Israeli poems. I presented one of these, "Yossi, My Successful Little Boy", in chapter two. It describes a mother who, seeking to perpetuate her son's love for her, accepts his basic lack of functioning and exalts him. The second poem, a sequel to this by a famous Israeli singer, Shlomo Artzi, contains an echo of the destructive results of this type of mothering. Intuitively the words describe how Yossi doesn't function in the army, but "stands like a Golem while others dash about", nor does he care about being like that. He is released from the army because of a psychological problem and is unable to find a wife. His mother "succeeded" in one of her various maternal tasks: she managed *not* to turn him into an Israeli combat fighter. Yossi ends up in an institution, hospitalized due to the inability for even minimal functioning. The poem ends with the mother's words repeated: "Yossi, my successful little boy."

Guilt is also a central component in parental relationships with their sons. This can be heard when the son blames the mother for turning him docile and obedient even when it comes to military instruction that could cause his death in the army.

I would like to emphasize that this parental dynamic can have a series of consequences, beginning with the possibility of military service suspending or severing parts of the maturation process. Military service may also create a "bubble" in which the adolescents adopt a false recruitment identity as though they are "playing at soldiering" and then find themselves in genuinely serious situations. There is also the possibility that during the encounter with the military system, the Israeli young man will open up traits he had been prevented from developing and will find an opportunity in military service to accelerate the maturation process and manifest the developmental messages of combat masculinity with all its various values that had been latent but, with recruitment, could take a front-row position.

There are many other questions related to these issues: Where does the son's identification with the father manifest even though the father, who is nonetheless a masculine combat figure, was silent? With whom do soldiers share their military experiences: mother, or father? What are the soldiers' perceptions of danger and fear? What are their plans for the future? Does the commander act as a kind of substitute father-figure since he is not silent but gives out commands, snubs his soldiers when necessary, but also makes sure they eat, sleep, and train well? What happens with sexuality in the army? Do humour and undignified rites-of-passage ceremonies provide cover for shame, distress, emotional inferiority? Where is violence directed—towards the enemy, the weakest one in the group unit, the youngest one?—and what does that lead to? What is the relationship between the group and the individual, when is loneliness felt, and are these feelings shared with mothers?

In chapter seven, I touch on the characteristics of the Israeli combatant over the generations and present additional information gained from discussions with soldiers who fought in a recent campaign.

Notes

1. I began conducting a study, in conjunction with the IDF, of the emotional processes undergone by the young Israeli from the moment he receives his first draft papers through his combat service. The research was interrupted by the Protective Edge War in Gaza (August 2014).

2. The practical analysis of results of parental conduct are presented in later chapters; the following analysis is of possible outcomes.

3. The issue of resolving the oedipal process in same-sex couples is too broad to be included in the current research in depth.

CHAPTER SEVEN

The warrior hero

. . . When you draw close this day to battle against your enemies, do not let your heart be faint, fear not nor be alarmed, and do not be frightened by them.

Deut. 20: 3

Cornerstones of the Israeli soldier's identity since 1948

Looking at the multiple layers of parenting sons in Israel and the couple-relationship patterns that develop, the parents' inter-generational baggage, as well as the emotional baggage of the sons themselves, two questions necessarily arise: "Who are you, Israeli soldier?" "How did the Israeli home, with all its unique facets, shape you?"

This chapter aims to show non-Israeli readers more of who the person is behind the label of "Israeli soldier" and thereby also better understand the internal Israeli experience rather than that portrayed externally in the media.

Who are you, Israeli soldier?

The essence of the question, "Who are you, Israeli soldier?" conceals a premise that a collective identity derives from the accrual of the various personal and group identities. In other words, a "collective identity" is a reflection of the ethos and norms common in that society in any particular period.

The Israeli soldier's image is shaped through a unique fabric of interwoven emotional and cognitive factors. Their complex emotional world consolidates throughout their development, from the parental processes described so far, the background of the unique Jewish Israeli history of past generations, and the modern Israeli history of continuous coping with hostilities.

There are multiple facets of soldiers' identities accrued over the course of their lives.[1] In view of the complexity and importance of this issue, a separate study is needed, using psychoanalytic research methods, of the conscious and unconscious emotional processes undergone by the Israeli as he is growing up, through military service, and then becoming a functioning male in society. This chapter should therefore be considered an introduction which nonetheless offers several significant understandings that may arouse continued thought and discourse.

Historical background

Familiarization with the historical background behind the foundation of the State of Israel and the IDF is vital for understanding the character of the Israeli soldier and the myth surrounding the soldier in Israeli society.

The milestones presented here are personal choices drawn from the associative mythic chain on which I was raised: as the daughter of a mother who is a Holocaust survivor and a father whose family arrived in Israel more than two centuries ago. Had my family background been different, my chain of associations would surely have been different.

The first collective Zionist immigration to Israel took place in 1806 with the arrival, in their hundreds, of the disciples of Rabbi Elijah Kremer, more commonly known as the *Vilna Gaon* ["the luminary of Vilna"] (Ben-Ariea & Reiner, 2003).[2]

Jewish communities over the world preserved their identity and their connection with Israel for centuries, even though control over the land of Israel changed hands frequently—from Hellenists to Hasmoneans, Romans to Byzantians, Arabs, Mameluke Crusaders, the Ottoman Empire, and finally the British, who conquered the area in 1917. In 1922 the League of Nations provided Britain with a mandate to rule the area of Israel; the mandate included the Balfour Declaration of 1917, establishing a national home for the Jews in the land of Israel.

In 1947, following World War II and the genocide of over 6 million Jews in Europe, the United Nations declared the establishment of the

Jewish state for the Jewish people in the land of Israel—the State of Israel. Under David ben Gurion, the first prime minister, the independent organizations known as the *Hagana* ("defence") and the six *Palmach* brigades were assimilated into a single military force, the IDF, charged with the purpose of protecting Israel's existence.

Surrounded by hostile countries and terror regimes, Israel has been in a state of war ever since, even if not continuously, and though two peace treaties—with Egypt and with Jordan—hold to this day. With soldiers killed and families left bereaved, the emotional fallout has seeped into the parenting of sons.

An example of the role of past history in the shaping of modern Israel's military and soldiers was given by Colonel Eliezer Toledano at the ceremony marking handover of command in May 2013. He mentioned two major influences in his life: first, the 1903 pogroms in Kishinev, following false accusations that Jews in that town had murdered a Christian boy for religious rites, when, in the Czar's name forty-nine Jews were murdered, hundreds were injured, and thousands of homes and stores were destroyed; he stated that "Jews must be able to protect themselves" and directly linked this historic event to "the right of existence of paratroopers being inherent to their operational ability to quickly respond to any IDF request and protect the people of Israel wherever they live". Second, the image of his friend Nadav Milo, commander of a paratrooper squadron, killed in Lebanon in 1997; Nadav's example was "a true beacon of human majesty," he concluded.

Milestones of an army at war

In 1947,[3] following refusal by Arab countries to accept the UN General Assembly's plan by which the trans-Jordan area would be divided into two states—the Jewish state and an Arab state, with an international corridor—Arabs attacked an Israeli bus; five of its Jewish passengers were murdered, an act that was considered to mark the start of the War of Independence. Armies from six countries invaded Israel's territory, supported by attacks emanating from within Arab homes inside Israel, in the effort to eliminate the Jewish presence and thwart the UN decision to establish the State of Israel. Some 6,000 Israelis died: about half long-standing citizens, the others Jewish immigrants recently arrived from war-torn Europe.

In 1956, the Kadesh Operation—the Sinai War—began as a result of escalated hostilities by Egypt, including Arab commando groups (Fedayeen) invading Israel via Gaza, blocking the passage of Israeli ships through the Suez Canal, and nationalizing the Anglo-French canal company. A coalition of British, French, and Israeli forces conquered half of the Sinai Peninsula; three days later the IDF withdrew, and international forces took over.

The 1967 Six Day War followed the closure of the Straits of Tiran—a pre-emptive attack by Israel in reaction to specific threats and known plans for war against Israel by its Arab neighbours. The outcome, reached in just six days in an overwhelming Israeli victory, was the conquest of areas previously under Jordanian control; half of the Sinai Peninsula held by the Egyptians; and the Golan Heights, captured from Syria. Following the deep existential anxiety of an army that had not yet fought a comprehensive war, this sweeping victory led to euphoria. Minister of Defence Moshe Dayan, already recognized as a war hero as Chief of Staff in the Sinai War, became a symbol of the hero who integrates military might and initiative, on the one hand, and deep roots in Israel's history, on the other.

The 1969 War of Attrition was instigated by Egypt to arouse opposition in the Israeli home front to continued occupation of Sinai.

At the 1972 Munich Olympics, the Palestinian Black September group slaughtered Israel's Olympic delegation of eleven athletes, trainers, and referees. The attackers were later tracked down and killed.

The 1973 Yom Kippur War, instigated by Egypt and Syria to retake the areas they lost in the Six Day War, broke out on the holiest day of the Jewish calendar, catching the IDF off-guard. In fact, Israel's government had ignored warnings that a war was brewing. Over 3,000 Israelis were killed during the war, and thousands were wounded or suffered shell shock. Following this war, Israel set up an investigative enquiry, the Agranat Commission, which found the military blameworthy, not the government. The crisis this war caused in Israeli society became evident only years later.

In 1976, an Air France flight from Israel to France, with 105 Jews, Israelis, and cabin crew on board, was hijacked by terrorists. In Operation Jonathan—the Entebbe Operation—in Uganda, all the terrorists were killed and almost all the kidnapped passengers and staff were saved—a major success for the IDF.

In 1979, a peace treaty was signed between Israel and Egypt. Prior to the signing, the Sinai Peninsula was returned to Egyptian control by Israeli forces. The treaty has held to date and currently includes cooperation between Israel and Egypt against the Hamas organization controlling Gaza.

In 1982, the *"Shlom Hagalil"* ("maintaining peace in the Galilee") war, intended as a limited operation to stop rockets being fired by the Palestine Liberation Organization (PLO) from southern Lebanon into northern Israel, quickly developed into a full-scale war, known as the First Lebanon War. Israel's government sought, unsuccessfully, to initiate a new order in Lebanon. A security strip was then created between Israel and southern Lebanon, and the PLO were driven out. For the first time the national consensus was split considerably—opposition, fierce political argument, and demonstrations peaked following the slaughter by Lebanese Christians of Lebanese Muslims in refugee camps under IDF responsibility. Although the war did cease formally, the IDF was dragged into securing that area of Lebanon for a further eighteen blood-shedding years. Only in May 2000 did all Israeli troops withdraw.

In 1987, the First Intifada (Arabic, "shaking off")—a predominantly violent uprising against Israeli rule of Palestinian residents in the West Bank and Gaza Strip—resulted in Israeli military personnel being killed and multiple terror attacks against civilians in Jerusalem. It ended with the signing of the 1993 Oslo Agreement.

In 1994, a peace agreement was signed between Jordan and Israel. Like the earlier agreement with Egypt, this peace treaty too has held. Jordan is also part of the coalition fighting Islamic extremism.

In 2000, the Second Intifada, marked by multiple suicide bombings against Israel's civilian population, resulted in expansion by Israel of its activities against terror organizations, in actions known as "targeted forestalments". Thousands of victims on both sides were the result. In 2002, in response to horrifying exhibitionist attacks, such as that in the packed Park Hotel dining hall in Netanya, the "Defensive Shield" operation destroyed terror cells in the Palestinian West Bank towns. A particularly harsh battle ensued in the Jenin refugee camp. In 2003, Arafat appointed Mahmoud Abbas (also known as Abu Mazen) as Prime Minister of the Palestinian Authority. A wave of terror attacks took place in cities across Israel. Abbas worked to achieve a *Hudna* (Arabic, "ceasefire")—a period of relative quiet, which nonetheless included terror attacks against Israeli civilians.

Despite massive opposition from inside and outside Israel, a security fence was erected separating Israel from the Palestinian territories, significantly reducing the number of attacks, particularly against Israeli West Bank settlements.

In 2000, following public opposition led by the "Four Mothers" organization (see chapter four), the IDF withdrew from all areas of

Lebanon, which included a narrow strip along the Lebanon–Israel border that had acted as a buffer against rocket attacks. With the IDF's fast exit from Lebanon, Hizbullah swiftly moved into the areas formerly held by the South Lebanon Army (SLA), which had cooperated with the IDF.

In 2005, the Gaza Strip was unilaterally evacuated by Israel; the IDF withdrew to the borders of "the green line". The plan was coordinated between Prime Minister Ariel Sharon and Mahmoud Abbas. At that time, the Gaza Strip contained the Fatah and Hamas organizations. In 2006/7 Hamas took control of Gaza, and Fatah of the West Bank.

In 2006, in reaction to the kidnapping by Hizbullah of two reservist soldiers, an operation was begun by the IDF, which turned into the Second Lebanon War. The war ended with the area being held by the SLA, with a UNIFIL (UN Interim Force in Lebanon) force along the border. Hizbullah lost some ten percent of its forces, but it rehabilitated bunkers throughout southern Lebanon and renewed its arsenal, including thousands of rockets smuggled out of Syria.[4] This operation disclosed multiple serious errors on the part of senior IDF ranks, as well as other severe failures and deficiencies. A public inquiry—the Winograd Commission—was appointed to examine all Lebanon-related issues.

In 2008, Operation Cast Lead followed incessant firing of rockets from Gaza Strip into Israel and the kidnapping of an Israeli soldier. Once its objectives had been reached, the operation was terminated, a unilateral ceasefire declared, and Israel exited Gaza.

In 2014, the huge Protective Edge Operation in Gaza was the response to renewed rocket fire from Gaza, with missiles approaching Tel Aviv.

This history of hostilities—often actual attacks on their and their families' lives—leads to the Israeli soldier's knowledge that he is directly protecting his own home. He is not going to war in the name of an ideology or to assist an ally, but to save the lives and homes of his family.

Israeli society is nonetheless split over the issue of Jewish towns built in areas conquered in the Six Day War. Some claim they are a hindrance to reaching a peaceful agreement with the Palestinians; others, that these towns throughout the West Bank protect Israel's heartland, allow ongoing contact with the Palestinian population, and maintain general peace. Some consider Israel's exit from Gaza in the interests of peace-seeking as political failure, with the area now a warren of underground terror bunkers—proving that building a stable peace is impossible.

Transformations in the Israeli soldier's image since Israel's establishment

The image of the Israeli soldier has undergone transformation over the generations, paralleling changes in the country itself. I shall look at six points in time: the War of Independence (1947), the Kadesh Operation (1956), the Six Day War (1967), the Yom Kippur War (1973), the Lebanon Wars (1985–2000), and Operation Protective Edge (2014).

The War of Independence

Three combatant identities can be characterized in the War of Independence, which was generally assigned a date of 1948 but actually took place between 1947 and 1949: soldiers born and bred in the land, Holocaust survivors from Europe, and non-Jewish volunteers from abroad.

The Israeli soldier of 1948 had nothing to lose. The soldier who came from the Holocaust had, in most cases, lost his entire family and experienced unimaginable cruelty. The soldier born and raised in Israel was conscious that his people had been exterminated in the Holocaust, and if he did not fight for his newly formed country, something similar may happen again. The Jews and the Arabs had been granted states by the United Nations: it was absolutely clear that the war was over the most basic right to exist.

According to Segev (2007), the War of Independence soldier is a *tzabar*: abrasive on the outside but soft and sensitive inside, a youth, a fighter, daring, rooted, ready to die protecting his home and family, willing to kill but cry over the death, a trusty comrade, disconnected from troubling doubts and from any real criticism. This image was primarily one of the Palmach fighter: young, daring, easy-going with mates, a strong fighter, brave, determined, professional, and willing to sacrifice his life without hesitation: bereavement is the constant partner of the figure of the 1948 soldier. At the same time, he is mischievous, a man who loves to play music and sing, a person with laughter in his eyes who loves being the focus of female admiration. "The Israeli soldier of '48 is one with a face and name, soldiers who are also people, soldiers who represent the new budding of the people" (Ofrat, 2004)—a description of the new spirit of spontaneity, creativity, initiative, and willingness for sacrifice. The soldier of that time, whose battle involved a good deal of improvisation, resourcefulness, derring-do, and no small amount of disorderliness, never internalized the concept of limits.

But this image of a figure of Israeli legend did not characterize the soldier who was an immigrant, a Holocaust survivor, or a Jewish refugee from an Arab country, forced to flee when Israel became a formal entity. This immigrant population was deemed inferior in both their motivation and their ability to fight (Lisak & Kimmerling, 1984). And, in fact, the Israeli reality of 1948 was different from the legend. A survey in 1949[5] found that, in contrast to the "romantic" perception of the War of Independence and the soldiers who fought in it, 70% of the overseas volunteers held negative opinions about the country, its population, and its military service. They noted that advancement is possible only through "*protekzia*"[6] and that the locals are inhospitable, unfriendly, impolite, insolent, and noisy. People are not interested in others' views, cannot stand that another person is occasionally right, and place too much importance on their country of origin. Lastly, they added that people in this country never rest and always claim they have no time.[7]

Israeli society was obviously unable to take a look at itself. It chose the image of the *tzabar* with brushed-back bangs as the symbol of the soldier, while the figure of the Diaspora Jew symbolized those who could be killed, like helpless sacrifices.

The maternal behavioural pattern found in this study, which pitches itself against the parts identified with their sons' combat masculinity, suggests that perhaps the difficulty in integrating conflictual parts has seeped into family relationships not just through complex emotional dynamics, but also through intergenerational transferring of this unresolved conflict, hence the need to identify the full range of facets of the Israeli personality and create a discourse between these and the characteristics of its behaviours, including those originally denied and suppressed.

The shared existential experience of the 1948 generation created the basic sense of shared destiny—values like comradeship, willingness to risk one's own life to save another's, love of the land, a commitment to life. Perhaps the purpose of the war—not only against the imminent danger of death but also towards establishing the state—caused libidinal and aggressive forces to be recruited in the psyches of soldiers with the goal of achieving this. When these two forces, which Freud explained as being conflictual in essence, are directed to the same place, they maximize the individual's power, for better or worse.

Integration of this nature can be found in Nathan Alterman's poem "The Silver Platter", which became a cornerstone of Israeli culture: it describes how, with the war clearly a victory, the nation faces its dead sons "donning celebration and horror", in a mixture of libidinal aggression. Asked in the poem who they are, they reply: "We are the silver platter on which the Jewish State is handed to you." This poem is still recited at military ceremonies and on memorial days, indicating the extent to which the soldier of today is shaped on the layers of identity from Israel's establishment. Ariel Hirschfeld, a researcher in Israeli literature and culture, opposed reading this poem,[8] decrying what he perceived to be its glorification and aestheticization of death. Perhaps unconsciously he felt that repeating these texts causes the trauma to be transmitted to coming generations.

The Kadesh Operation (Sinai War)

The 1956 Kadesh Operation reinforced the glorification of the warrior *tzabar* (Almog, 1997) and helps understand the current reality as addressing the destruction of the Jews by the Nazis, as explained by Professor Nathan Rotenstreich:

> We are proud of the army which symbolizes the end of our dependence on protection provided to us, miserable and persecuted, by foreigners, and because it manifests one of the discoveries that we can stand up for ourselves. [in Bar-On, 1999]

The public view between the Sinai War and the Yom Kippur War identifies the representative soldier in the elite group as linking directly with ancient forefathers, the soldier leaders Joshua bin-Noon and King David (Hadari, 2002). Present and past are intertwined in one historical continuity moving in the opposite direction. It is not as though the giving of the Torah (Bible) led to the Sinai War, but the Sinai War establishes Mount Sinai's Biblical role. Unlike chronological time, which moves forward, time in this case moves backwards. The conquest of Sinai is no longer a tactical action aimed at opening the Straits of Tiran but a return to the Revelation at Mount Sinai.

The Six Day War

Following the sweeping victory of the 1967 Six Day War, we encounter a different soldier. The young commanders of 1948, now in their late forties or early fifties, are military leaders (see chapter five).[9] The figure of the Israeli soldier of the Six Day War is a marvellous hero who succeeded not only in saving the country from extinction and paralysing the enemy forces in just six days, but also expanded the country's borders and, most importantly, freed Jerusalem, including the ancient Western Wall, the last remnant of the Second Temple, destroyed in 70 CE. In actuality, this soldier is the epitome of the image of 1948's *tzabar*.

Unforgettable images and voices are engraved in the collective Israeli memory: the photograph of a paratrooper crying at the Western Wall; the handsome soldier raising his gun at the Suez Canal on the cover of *Time* magazine; Motta Gur's declaration on reaching the Wall that "The Temple Mount is in our hands!"; the speech at the Mount of Olives by then Chief of Staff Yitzhak Rabin, stressing the IDF's values of comradeship, spirit, and courage.

The disparity between the tremendous existential anxiety before the war and the swift victory was so huge that the war was seen as miraculous, its generals and soldiers blindly admired. Victory albums flourished, generals were celebrated on game cards, calendars, postcards, etc. The encounter with "the city of the fathers" in general, and with the Old City of Jerusalem in particular, began to sprout a messianic approach and a sense of Third Temple kingship. During that period, the book *The Tanks of Tammuz* (Teveth, 1968) became a ritualized symbol of boastful admiration towards the generals, the headiness of power, and scorn of the enemy.[10]

The return of a threat to the country's very existence, followed by the enemy's crushing defeat, undoubtedly raises the emotional content of Holocaust trauma, as though recurring in the present, with the establishment of the state being the solution that saves the people. This dynamic is reinforced and embedded in the conscious and unconscious levels simultaneously, as expressed in Yitzhak Rabin's Mount of Olives speech detailing the tremendous excitement sweeping through the troops, the paratroopers who freed the Western Wall leaning against it and crying, the deep sense of relief, the fear that preceded their conquest, and the sense of spiritual revelation in Jewish history's battles.[11]

Once again, as in 1948, other voices were left in the shadows, and opinions expressing the price of the war were presented as contradicting the fervent reaction to victory. A group of soldiers from the kibbutz movement found it hard to join in the euphoria (Shapira, 1967). As Avishai Grossman said: "A lack of joy typifies those of us returning from the war. I don't have the feeling that this was the last time that those living here will put on their uniforms" (in Gan, 2009).

In his Mount of Olives speech, Yitzhak Rabin related to these young adults with a lack of understanding:

> More and more we come across a strange phenomenon among our fighters. They cannot be fully happy, and a good measure of sorrow and shock mingle with their celebrations, while others do not celebrate at all. Our warriors on the front lines saw . . . not only the glory of victory but also its price: comrades fell alongside them. And I know the terrible price paid by the enemy which weighs deeply. . . . Perhaps the Jewish people were not educated and accustomed to feeling the joy of conquest and victory. This is why the matter is received with mixed feelings.

In the public's mind, as in the collective memory, the combatants' discourse was engraved as the manifestation of the "shoot but cry" image representing those "good yet tormented souls" with troubled consciences over the cruelty arising from the act of war (Teveth, 1968).

Hadari (2002) identified every difficulty or anxiety being experienced in Israeli society as depression, and every victory as euphoria.

Tom Segev (2007) also found that there was no justification for the sense of loss prior to the war, nor for the euphoria afterwards, because the conquests of 1967 occurred despite government decisions, and the generals used too much force and escalated the crisis (Teveth, 1968).

The Yom Kippur War

Pervasive complacency following the Six Day War exacted a high price in the 1973 Yom Kippur War, which caught Israel unawares and unprepared. Once again an entire country found itself clouded in gloom, rife with existential anxiety, but this time there were no stories of easy victory—on the contrary: despite ultimately prevailing, the IDF absorbed massive losses.

The warriors of the Yom Kippur War—the sons of those who fought the War of Independence—had been youths at the time of the Six Day War just six years earlier. But their experience was the opposite of the narratives on which they were raised. The threat to Israel's existence was real and severe, but the military in which they served was neither professional nor prepared. Victories were achieved only with luck and despite mishaps, faulty equipment, and casualties from "friendly fire" (Levi, 2003).

Following this war, the feeling in the country was harsh. The conclusions of the Agranat Commission shook the foundations of the state, much as the war itself had done, with the bulk of the blame placed on the military leaders. The government resigned, top-ranking commanders were demoted, and the IDF began a massive rehabilitation phase, simultaneous to legislative and intelligence adjustments.

In Shmuel Schnitzer's words:

> . . . absolute confidence in the leadership no longer exists. There are no more infallible leaders, there are no more national heroes who can be utterly relied upon . . . there is no absolute respect for any body or any state institution. The public . . . has learned to use its judgement much more than before. Politics has ceased to be a matter for politicians and security no longer a matter only for generals. . . . The population wants to know the facts, examine the motives, hear the reasoning. [*Maariv*, 25 June 1982]

The war had deepened anxiety over annihilation and shattered the illusions around security, rousing the nation from its torpor.

Schnitzer described an integrative state of mind—the opposite of those fully in the know versus those who know nothing, total heroes who can blindly and confidently be followed. The issue, in psychoanalytic terms, is whether this was a transition from a paranoid-schizoid attitude that splits good and bad into a depressive attitude—which, despite the word used to describe it, is actually a healthy state that comprehends outcomes of lack of success as being an integration of positive and negative factors—or a transition from the other side of the coin: replacement of the manic experience by the opposite experience of despair, as described by Hadari (2002).

Accordingly, the surplus parental anxiety we found in the research, unconsciously transferred to the sons, may result from the parents' experiences as soldiers in the Yom Kippur War or as youths who understood what happened. When David (see chapter three) shared his feelings of deep fear when setting out on a mission and the fact that some will not return, saying it may be impossible to prepare for such an experience, he related both to the Yom Kippur War and the two Lebanon wars that followed.

It is important to examine what replaced the "rescue (saviour?) fantasy" that disappeared: a realistic evaluation of the situation, including its strengths and weaknesses, or the terrifying anxiety of the warrior in a harsh war?

During the 1970s and 1980s, the image of the Israeli soldier changed in Israeli art, expressing its demythologization: no women appeared in artwork with soldiers, and there is disharmony between the soldiers and nature. There are dead soldiers, as in paintings by Pamela Levi or Avishai Eyal, and blood, as in Moshe Gershoni's paintings. The victim's pathos is replaced by the generalness of the sprawled body (Ofrat,

2004). In 1991, soldiers' features are virtually obliterated, their identities generalized, technological, anonymous. Emphasis is on turning "the individual cadet into a war machine". Ofrat notes that the image of the soldier in his helmet, holding his Uzi, leaning against the Western Wall, expresses the secularization of the soldier and his alienation from the thrilling religious context. But in this image one can also see the brilliant figure of the man of our times—the Israeli man in particular.

The First and Second Lebanon Wars

From the 1980s through the early 2000s, the Israeli soldier fought terror organizations in the West Bank, Gaza Strip, and Lebanon. The First Lebanon War, which began in 1982, was the first perceived by the public as a war of choice, its goal being to combat the PLO's attacks from within Lebanon. There was, for the first time, a lack of consensus in the Israeli public relative to war. Soldiers often felt unsupported by the public. The Israeli soldier found himself in depressive policing roles over the Lebanese civilian population—a task almost unequalled for igniting the political awareness of young people who were simultaneously being harmed by the disruption to their civilian lives (Levi, 2003). On the part of the Israeli public, absolute identification with the goals of war was replaced by ambivalence. The IDF was perceived as carrying out military procedures the necessity or outcomes of which were disputed.[12] It was also perceived as, at the least, turning a blind eye to the massacre in the refugee camps. The disparity between political and military goals also caused conflict in Israeli society.

There was, for the first time, no unequivocal backing by the public of the *tzabar* soldier image. Moreover, the tension between the *tzabar* and the immigrant who had experienced the Holocaust was identifiable within the government. Minister of Defence Ariel Sharon—symbol of the *tzabar* soldier, undisciplined, unruly—pushed for increasingly expansive actions; Prime Minister Menachem Begin, whose only goal was to distance the threat from the country's borders, accused Sharon of lying. Following numerous demonstrations, a government investigative committee's conclusions led to the replacement of Ariel Sharon and the rebuking of Rafael Eitan, chief of staff at the time.

"A soldier who's emotionally scarred or hurt . . . is a national problem, that's clear to us", said Brigadier General Ben Yishai, implying that the home front can no longer bear death but only the lightest of casualties, according to the description he gave to reporter Ilana Dayan. At the same time he described his love of action, which requires alertness, creativity, and constant tension. Dayan, who had been with the fighters in Lebanon, identified "Lebanon fear" on their faces. Soldiers active in the Second Lebanon War had been toddlers at the time of the First Lebanon War.

The Sabra and Shatilla massacre

In September 1982, during the Lebanon Civil War, the Christian Phalangists massacred hundreds of refugees in the Palestinian refugee camps of, predominantly, Sabra and Shatilla, in West Beirut. Thousands of Palestinian fighters were rumoured to be hiding in the camps, so the IDF avoided entering these and the Phalangist forces went in instead. Following a public outcry, a government commission found no proof of direct IDF involvement in the massacre, but that at some point IDF commanders knew of events and took no decisive steps to intervene. Strong criticism was levelled at the leadership of the IDF.

Numerous songs, poems, and films explored the massacre, among them the award-winning animated documentary film *Waltz with Bashir*, through which the director, Ari Folman, struggles to recall and digest, twenty-five years after the events, his experiences as an Israeli soldier in 1982. In conversations with a friend who suffers from recurring nightmares connected with the refugee camps even though he can't recall ever being there, he himself eventually faces his own truth without dissociation and remembers firing off flares over the refugee camps that night. For this, he feels guilty. He finally realizes that he had witnessed a massacre under the Israeli soldiers' very noses.

The film character, Ari, tries to cope with the integrated layer of powerfully awakening libidinal aggression. The film met with mixed reactions, some claiming that yet again it presents the image of the IDF victim. Herzliya Mayor Eli Landau claimed, in contrast, that "the film opposes the State of Israel . . . since it also places blame on our shoulders for cooperating with the massacre in the refugee camps, which is a total lie".

It is evident that Ari Folman attempts, through the medium of film, to process and symbolize his harsh experiences of Lebanon. However, perhaps that same dynamic of cohesion between anxiety, aggression, and the pleasure of powerful drives too difficult to contain exacts the price that Bion (1959) describes as "an attack on linking": damage to cogitation and the ability for moral thinking.

French philosopher Jean Baudrillard (1981) explains how postmodern culture finds difficulty in preserving the connection between speech and language, and reality, which gives rise to a simulacrum[13]—the factor that exists between the representation (the symbolized) and the word (the symbol) that disturbs the processes of representation. This blocks the sense of truth and leads to every cultural discourse being movement between empty representations. In such a state, there is constant mourning and purposelessness, which creates a pretence of self-consciousness.

Ashkenazi (2010) claimed that this is precisely what occurs in Folman's film: focus on the soldier's trauma while ignoring the suffering of the other side. The victim is the Israeli soldier, exposed to harsh events: it is he who is shown to suffer nightmares, anxiety, and post-traumatic stress disorder (PTSD) as a result, rather than the true victims of the war—the Lebanese soldiers and civilians.

The following examples give further testimony to the understanding of how emotional charges of the past and the present mix. The pogroms of Kishinev and the genocide of the Holocaust relative to the Sabra and Shatilla massacre find expression in Mira Ravikovitch's poem "A Baby Can't Be Killed Twice". Perhaps it echoes a line in a poem by Haim Nahman Bialik, "On Slaughter", written about the 1903 Kishinev pogroms: "Revenge for the small child's blood has not been created yet by Satan." In a poem following the Sabra and Shatilla massacre, Amnon Dankner writes: "I saw, I heard, and there is no end for victims and killing" (quoted in Hever & Ron, 1983); the poem opens with a description of soldiers sitting around for two days, "Not seeing not hearing Without eyes, ears. That's how the Jewish soldier sits." The work ends: "And for more than a generation's span the images will pursue us—Of those lying in alleys and the slaughtered in the camps

Vamık Volkan (2012) noted that this process also comes about in moments of deadlock in negotiations between enemy countries, when intergenerational trauma is raised repeatedly as a way of justifying the situation, instead of seeking renewed creative thinking. Tal (1991, cited in Ashkenazi, 2010) found the same in his study of trauma among Vietnamese soldiers: trauma as the substitute for every moral discourse became a tool that permits every moral action in the view of soldier and public, blocking the ability to hold to the stance of considering and observing—a reflexive position that enables symbolization, mentalization, and the vital emotional processing needed to release the present from preventing the reconstruction of historic traumatic charges.

At the close of millennium, soldiers were represented in art from a critical perspective as operatives of a controversial policy. Admittedly, young artists did depict anti-militarist and anti-macho figures, and some expressed a homoerotic military reality. It is also possible to identify components of parental guilt in sending their sons to their death through the army. David Tartakover portrayed the soldier alongside a mother and called the artwork "Mother". Avishai Eyal painted dead soldiers at the feet of elderly mothers, highlighting the idea that the dissonance between the soldier and the mother is greater than the harmony between them. Ivan Schwebel painted himself in the role of King David, with his soldier-son in the role of the biblical Uriah; the message is one of betrayal by a father who sends his soldier-son to his death (Ofrat, 2004). Israeli art is apparently manifesting the emotional processes found in this study.

Examining changes in the portrayal of the Israeli soldier from 1948 to 2009 via images from the journal *Bamakhaneh*,[14] Efrat Shalvi (2016) found that the image did not change from one form to another, but developed with increasing complexity, an additional image being added from one period to another, creating a complex and highly developed image of the combat soldier. Shalvi describes this development as being linked, among other things, to social changes at the national level, such as the "Four Mothers" organization (see chapter two), whose activities infused the military discourse with an attitude towards soldiers as "our children", blurred the boundaries between private and public space, and brought women's voices into a public military space that had been closed to them previously. The image of the combatant altered from being an emotionless killing machine in the military space to a soldier who also takes up private familial space and expresses various emotions that do not detract from his ability to be a "war machine". In the early 2000s, for example, additional layers are ascribed to the soldier of the humane occupation army that reacts generously to the Palestinian population and expresses emotion through physical contact, or pain through tears, etc. These findings are consistent with the understanding that the process undergone by the Israeli soldier is a transition from a stance in which the dynamic of splitting between good and bad is the controlling stance, to one of an integrative emotional dynamic in which there is room for both the brave parts and the soft parts. Simultaneously, mothers begin to appear in photographs of soldiers—a phenomenon that is consistent with findings of this study.

In the early twenty-first century, the Israeli soldier seems to have become humanized, lifted out of automatic military isolation—a human individual entity on the one hand and a manipulative ironic entity on the other. A work by a female sculptor in an art exhibition in Tel Aviv consisted of a bench with all of a soldier's personal equipment, embroidered with delicate beading that displays mythological figures of a world that is all good—an image that accords with the complex messages surfacing in this study, and detailed particularly in chapter two, on maternal conduct.

In the First Intifada, which commenced in 1987, and again in the Second Intifada of 2000, the Israeli soldier found himself facing an uprising of a wild multitude, and of terrorists. During these periods, soldiers continued to be related to as "our children", and the conflict surfaced between the actions expected of them and the values on which they had been raised. Yitzhak ben Aaron, for example, stated that the Israeli population seemed unaware of the dilemma facing their children: sent on impossible missions, using weapons against people throwing stones, yet expected to behave liberally and ethically in hate-ridden and violent situations. They are the victims of policy—not just the government's, but their parents', in their own home (quoted in Zilberstein, 2013).

The Israeli soldier serving during the intifada period did indeed occasionally feel clear dissonance between his values and his actions. Liebes and Blum-Kulka (1994) analysed soldiers' accounts of their experiences and found they employed several coping patterns by cognitive reorganization through structuring frameworks that reduce the inconsistency, justify obedience, improvise behaviours, negotiate with external reality, and separate the action from the sensations and feelings—summed up by the researchers as shooting being one thing and weeping another.

However, they also found that sometimes, when the ego was required to cope with opposing actions, some voluntarily preferred not to avoid the pain created by the dissonance. In my view, this transition, from the fashionable experience of shooting to the fashionable experience of weeping, might indicate an important ability to transition between different emotional states rather than pathological splitting. The ability to talk about the conflict and the dissonance, and to move between contradictory emotional states, expresses the Israeli soldier's developing capacity to be in an integrative emotional state[15] rather than adapting himself to a unidimensional state, as in earlier wars.

Operation Protective Edge, Summer 2014

Operation Protective Edge ended while I was writing this chapter. For fifty days, southern Israel was pounded by rockets and missiles launched from the Hamas-ruled Gaza Strip. Following the kidnapping of three Israeli teenagers by Hamas operatives, a campaign opened initially under the banner of "Bring Our Boys Back", though it shortly became clear that the youths had been murdered. Israel increased its air attacks against Hamas's terrorist infrastructure. Israel's Iron Dome anti-missile system destroyed long-range missiles launched by Hamas, thereby preventing thousands of civilian deaths. Penetration by thirteen Hamas terrorists into Kibbutz Zikim in Israel's south via underground tunnels led to the IDF's entry into Gaza proper to destroy both the vast number of Hamas tunnels dug into southern Israel and as much of Hamas's arsenal as possible. The continual air-raid sirens, the dash to bomb shelters, and the exploding missiles drew Israelis into unity and broad support for the military action, combined with determination and robustness on the home front. This feeling altered somewhat after the government agreed to an "arrangement" that included a ceasefire but was viewed as not resolving the very foundations of problem.

Outlines of the 2014 Israeli soldier's image

It is possible to identify common outlines for the image of the 2014 Israeli soldier that echo the conscious and unconscious motifs and patterns detailed in earlier chapters. However, a more accurate image is possible only with some distancing from the events, to allow a broader perspective. The content below may therefore be "contaminated" by emotional defences such as rationalization, a psychic procedure in which the subject tries to provide a logical, consistent, or accepted explanation from the ethical perspective for stances, actions, ideas, emotions, etc. for which the true motives are impossible to perceive (Laplanche & Pontalis, 1973).

Today we encounter a soldier very different from the ones characterizing the earlier milestones. On the one hand, Israeli society still embraces and praises its soldiers, particularly those in combat units. On the other hand, something basic has changed in the attitude towards military service. Materialism is more pronounced, part of the search for an easier life; tolerance towards loss of life has dropped, as well as willingness to pay that price (Harel, 2013), as seen in the interviews.

The army no longer enforces combat service on cadets, nor remaining in combat units throughout military service, as it did in the past;

joining elite combat units is voluntary, and a recruit may be offered several options. A halo of prestige has been added to roles that do not involve any danger, such as the IDF's cyber unit (Harel, 2013). All this is known to mothers who tried diverse manipulations towards directing the sons they were raising to such units.

The soldier of 2014 has experienced war and knows it can break out again at any moment. Even those who have not actually fought have tangible experience of its existence and know that at any moment they might find themselves fighting.

Freud (1915c) admitted that his knowledge of the changes occurring in the soldier's psychology was very limited and that investigating this field was important. I shall try to begin that study here and ascertain what happens in the psyche of the soldier of 2014 who has experienced military service under routine circumstances in times of relative quiet, and in real war. Several sources were available to me: interviews I conducted with two soldiers who had just returned from Operation Protective Edge in Gaza; three recorded interviews with reservists who had also fought in Gaza (available on the Israeli news website Ynetnews); a text by a soldier who fought in Gaza written in between returning home on weekends and participating in a theatre workshop for soldiers; and Amos Harel's (2013) interviews with soldiers currently training as combatants, with their commanders, and with the soldiers' parents. Psychoanalytic insights shed light on recurring emotional processes in soldiers' experiences. I hope that these thoughts will become the basis for a deeper study into the concealed layers of the psyche of the young Israeli as he becomes a combat soldier, and after his discharge from the army.

Transitioning from adolescent identity to combatant identity

Recruitment occurs at age eighteen, during late maturation. Maturation completes the genital stage from the perspective of psycho-sexual development (Blos, 1962). Physiological changes bring about psychic changes. New instinctive drives appear and alter the ego's previous structure (A. Freud, 1936). The adolescent, seeking to adapt to these developmental changes as part of consolidating his unique separate identity, redefines himself through psychic reorganization. The environment assists in attributing new meanings to the reorganization and repression of the self as the adolescent undergoes a complex interpersonal process of compromise between his personal interests and the possibilities offered by the environment. This process requires reorganization of the self while preserving enough of the authentic self in the adolescent's changing world (Slavin & Kriegman, 1992).

Most teenagers in the Western world undergo this process in a civilian environment, whereas for the Israeli teen it takes place in a military environment. Straight from the protective home environment that typifies senior school, where efforts are directed at making life easier and more pleasant for boys, the teens enlist and need to adopt a military identity in which the central value is the myth of heroism, the ability to resist pain and display omnipotence and toughness (Lieblich, 1989; Sasson-Levy, 2006).

Experiences such as complete devotion among the soldiers and the idealization by one's family and the larger society may serve as facilitating factors for development. However, it may be inhibited within the army by reduced possibilities for social experimentation, dependency, and lack of direct emotional contact with females (Yerushalmi, 1997).

The multitude of elements involved in military service—from the trivial, such as discipline, type of nutrition, and physical prowess, to values, responsibility, personal challenge, solidarity—all work to shape the soldier's development and adult identity. The process takes place through training the cadet to assimilate discipline by isolating him from civilian life, subjecting his will to that of his commanders, undergoing processes of de-civilization and de-individualization through tough attitudes and punishment that cause regression, but also dependency and undisputed obedience, which is attained by providing compensatory rewards (Shatan, 1977). The military therefore becomes tremendously responsible towards the individual who enlists, and towards the entire society.

Sasson-Levy (2006) found that the developmental thirst for individuality and masculinity drives the adolescent to fully adopt the military-combat image, because the combat identity emphasizes personal ability, autonomy, achievement, and self-realization. Together, self-control and thrill create an individualized self-perception (Sasson-Levy, 2006)—traits that had encountered resistance by the mother, backed up by the father's silence, during the adolescent's development.

The newly recruited young man must bridge the disparity between how he knows himself as an adolescent in his protective home life, and learning about himself through the exhausting training that will turn him into a combat soldier. Israeli society acknowledges the difficult transition from home life to military life, as manifested by the popularity of military preparation courses and other such initiatives. The main focus is on the physical aspect, building stamina and fitness, but there are also leadership exercises, familiarization with the IDF, field days, first aid, field navigation, etc. These undoubtedly reduce the shock value of the transition to military service. Little is done, however, in relation to psychological readiness.

I feel that because we barely relate to the process undergone by these young men before they become combat soldiers, we leave them alone with all they undergo. The difficulties, however, create the use of defence mechanisms on the axis marked, at one pole, by avoidance and disregard, through denial and repression, and all the way at the other to a dissociative state in which it is impossible to know that the process is even occurring.

Support for the new recruit is often found among his peers, with whom he undergoes processes of socialization and "mirroring" confirmation. In the family, however, it often seems that the anxiety felt by parents makes things harder for the young man.

Mothers interviewed in this study intervened frequently as a means of directing their sons' lives, making it harder for the latter to achieve separation and individuation. The fathers enable this dynamic to occur by remaining silent, which skirts the issue. This type of conduct continues even after the son has enlisted. In his *feuilleton* "His Parents", Efraim Sidon describes the Israeli child's parents "Breathing down his neck and hot on his heels, behind him, alongside him, everywhere around him": even if he's a battalion commander, pilot, scientist, or inventor, he has no chance of escape, especially none from "the Jewish mother". Congruent with the insights arising from this study, Sidon identifies the parental conduct, but also focuses the perspective it contains that sets into action the emotional and behavioural dynamic, "the Jewish mother".

In *Every Hebrew Mother Will* (2013), Amos Harel described participating in and documenting meetings between parents and Nahal Brigade commanders throughout the sons' training in cadet camp. The interviews he conducted with parents and soldiers allow us to get an "insider" picture of this aspect of Israeli soldiering, and it is possible to identify parental patterns found in our study continuing into the army too, and to evaluate their impact on these sons-soldiers. We can also try to identify how the maturation and individuation process occurs despite difficulties arising from parental patterns.[16]

Some mothers identified their sons' entry into primary school as paralleling recruitment and arousing the same emotional elements of anxiety and hostile behavioural pattern towards systems that "take our son for themselves" and "might harm him". Harel's impression was that parents' attitudes were annoying, whining, and not to the point. One of the mothers, a teacher, identified the similarity between the parents' attitude towards the Nahal Brigade commanders and the attitude of parents at her school and described them as "nuisances" (Harel, 2013).

Mothers functioning as the trumpet of anxiety, and their attitude towards the young man enlisting as a "boy", are duplicated with the soldiers and families that Harel met, but it seems that there, despite the mother continuing her efforts at being dominant, the father was sometimes less silent, and the anxiety was shared between both parents. For example, Noy stated that his father, who served in the Nahal Brigade and fought in the Yom Kippur War, "reacted fine" with his choice of Nahal, but it was difficult for his mother. The very fact that soldier-sons express this themselves indicates that the uncontained maternal anxiety has been transmitted onto the sons' shoulders.

Parental feelings of guilt were expressed when, in an effort to remove their guilt relative to "should anything happen to him", they stressed that their son himself decided to enlist into a combat unit. Harel described how Tamir, whose elective subject for matriculation was computer studies, rejected offers to join a cyber unit, preferring instead to go into an infantry brigade. He is named for his uncle, who was killed in the First Lebanon War and also served in the Nahal Brigade. Tamir remembered how soldiers from the brigade came to the memorial ceremonies and would say: "When you're big, come and join Nahal." Tamir's father recognized his son's masculine combat characteristics, noting that his son serves in a combat unit "yet he doesn't complain". Tamir's mother, in contrast, spoke about her son as though referring to an unprotected small child: it is worth keeping in mind that the situation was cadet training, not real wartime. She maintained *daily* contact with Tamir and acknowledged that she invades his privacy by "checking when he goes on WhatsApp . . . I really can't understand how parents and soldiers managed in the days before mobile phones".

Compared to the silence of fathers in our study, where no acknowledgment is made of the sons' maturation and sexuality, leaving the space wide open to maternal takeover, here the father does acknowledge his son's maturation when Tamir comes home. Perhaps that is what allowed Tamir's mother, over whom Tamir towers, to smile and join in with this acknowledgment: "He's become a man."

Is the mother's ability to accept her son's masculinity connected to the father's entry into the picture? In other words, did the entry of the third—the father to the mother–son dyad—allow the mother to acknowledge her son's maturation on its way to the oedipal resolution?

Harel described a similar dynamic occurring in another part of the military base. Itamar enlisted a few months after his brother Amit was discharged, at the rank of battalion commander. Like other mothers in this study, Itamar's mother manifested the conflict she felt between her clear, unequivocal stance relative to the need to serve and the anxiety that had filled her from when he was born. And indeed, she teased him as though not seriously acknowledging him as a real soldier in the IDF: "You look like 'The Good Soldier Schweik', with your uniform falling off you." Itamar tried to show her he was no child and is coping well with the demands of cadetship, saying that he surprises himself with his abilities and even enjoys the training. But she does not forego her control, and on her way to check the tent he sleeps in, she "plasters a kiss on Commander Caspi's cheek" because her oldest son had once been Caspi's commander—as though declaring that she does not respect or accept her son's masculinity, nor that of her son's commander, who himself had been under her oldest son's command.

Here, too, the father did not remain silent but cynically shot back: "In the end they probably get a key ring." He added that when he served, there had been no such thing as "Parents' Day". No parent checked up on commanders or told them what was allowed or forbidden. There was no audit committee on treatment of cadets, parents did not phone commanders, and all equipment was supplied by the army and through recruits' own initiatives: unlike today, where parents purchase—sometimes in exaggerated quantities—whatever their sons need. He summarized: "They've crossed the line of reasonableness, and let parents interfere. An army can't be run by parents" (Harel, 2013, p. 197).

The reaction of both fathers raises the need to examine whether, after recruitment, they adopt a more active role with regard to mothers and sons.

Just days after the war ended, I met Ido, aged twenty and serving in the tanks corps, and his friend Ziv, aged twenty-one, serving in the combat engineering unit. They were still strongly tied to their impressions of the war, trying to digest what had happened, what is happening, and what could happen. They had fought in the first wave of military entering Gaza.

One of the first topics both raised was the frustration and harsh consequences of parental pampering and intervention and its effect on soldiering, demonstrating the outcomes of an attitude of protectiveness and leniency. Ido said, without even being prompted:

> "In training it happens all the time, parents are really protective of their kids, call the commanders up because of some penalty their kid got. When we were in cadet training in the firing field, I happened to overhear my commander talking with a really pressured mother. But the kids are simply . . ."

And then he corrected "kids":

> ". . . the soldiers don't have their phones with them, so she called him and said 'What? My kid? He doesn't have his phone? I can't get hold of him for four days already.' . . . The commander said to her: 'Lady, everything's fine, your kid doesn't need to talk to you right now. Bye.'"

Ziv also related to the same issue:

> "All the army's got this thing where parents complain . . . to the commander above the direct commander, and he then gets penalized . . ."

Ido added that it also affects training. Ziv said:

> "The army is so afraid you'll get hurt, or something will happen to the soldiers, that they don't let you train up and learn. Let's say there's . . . this type of sharpshooters' weapon, its large and used to blow up explosives from a distance. Even though in the war the guy with this weapon had to use it several times, before the war he hadn't even once . . . they're so afraid something will happen that the guy never even practised with this weapon.
>
> Or . . . in the war, when you get to a building, you connect the explosives together, stand behind it at a safe distance, and blow it up. But in training, to make sure there's no danger and no one will get hurt, you practise with all the materials disconnected, and then it's not realistic."[17]

Ido identified the source of that situation in discipline issues among soldiers, and the commanders' tied hands arising from parental intervention and their exaggerated protectiveness.

> "This excess carefulness derives from not relying enough on soldiers' discipline during training. And also because parents are so overprotective towards their children. For example, when their child gets punished in a way that seemed to them a bit out of proportion, they straight away contact the senior commander. Then he comes down on the lower-level direct commander who gave the punishment. Then the lower-level commander won't punish the soldier, because he doesn't want to get punished himself . . . then the soldier understands what's going on and won't respect the discipline . . . As a commander, you can't give out punishment, you can hardly do anything to punish your soldier . . . If you can't train properly, then in the battle you get hit . . ."

Ido and Ziv darted in and out of each other's remarks and together said:

> "And it creates problems because . . . they understand what the commander's allowed to do and what the commander's forbidden to do, and they take advantage of it . . . Then when the commander demands they do more, the soldier later sets him up and snitches on him to the senior commanders.
>
> In the war it was different . . . there, full support was given . . . but outside that there isn't full support, you need to . . . make sure you don't go beyond your authority even the smallest bit because otherwise they can set you up . . . I'm not saying it's like that everywhere. In some places the senior ranks . . . really support their staff, but *when that doesn't happen, it's terrible, because you have no firm ground to rely on."*

Ido demonstrated how this problem damages the ability to rely on other soldiers:

> "We're the soldiers raised on cream. It creates a situation where all kinds of guys who are supposedly fighting and should be ready for this, aren't. In the end, when you get down to brass tacks, you say to yourself, 'I don't want to be with so-and-so in the battle. Sure, he completed the training, but I don't want to be with him in the war because I don't think he can take the action.'"

The feeling that surfaces from Ido's and Ziv's descriptions is that among the ranks the sense of "a scale of fear" runs like a silken thread, where the person with authority is under threat from his cadets via orchestrating parents. The feeling is reinforced by the fact that, post-war, national and international investigative commissions passed judgement on commanders and soldiers. Ido talked about how that affected them:

> "You're afraid of it, after going into action, because every small mistake the IDF makes, you feel like you're being looked at as though you're not okay."

Harel notes how the protective mothering pattern that pampers and intervenes also manifests in the conversations between commanders and parents—as when Captain Naomi Caspi, commander of the November 2011 recruits said to parents: "Before the army your *child* used to sleep eighteen hours a day." The commander did not use the term "soldier" or even "today's soldier, when he was a child" but links himself to the infantile attitude shown by parents towards soldiers.

The same was true at a meeting I attended some several years ago between parents of combat soldiers and the leading IDF command. Chief of Staff Dan Halutz opened the event by saying, "Your children are our children"; the other generals followed with similar remarks. In hours of conversation about the current and future service of these soldiers, the word "soldier" was never used, only various forms of "child".

Remarks made by Ido and Ziv showed their intense need for a commander who arouses confidence, one who could be followed "through fire and water", who would prepare them fully for war and give them confidence in their ability to achieve their goals while nonetheless guarding their lives. Freud explained that in large groups there is a need for a strong authority figure, an admired "great commander" to submit to, be dominated by, and sometimes even suffer for; it is based on the longing for the father nested inside us. He is the father who, in legend, the hero is proud to have defeated: decisive, powerful, self-reliant, to the point of thoughtless oblivion. It is the hero who can be admired and trusted and always arouses awe (Freud, 1939, pp. 129–130). Like the great commander, the great leader impacts the people through personality and the idea for which she or he fights. The idea can emphasize an old concept existing in the hearts of the populace, or present a purpose based on a new concept (Freud, 1939). If this holds true for everyday life, how much more so in situations involving life-endangering battles.

We have seen how, in the Israeli constellation, fathers found difficulty in representing this image for their sons, and perhaps the absence of childhood intensifies the need for freedom. It comes as a surprise to find how the mother's dominant place, and parental difficulty in setting boundaries for their sons, confronting them with difficulties and conflicts in their attempts to create a reality in which happiness is the leading value, has seeped into the military.

Compared to the attitude glorifying the image of the soldier since the establishment of Israel, as detailed at the start of this chapter, treating soldiers not as fighting men but as "mama's little boys" causes a "clear drop in the degree of willingness on Israeli society's part to accept the death of soldiers as an inseparable, unavoidable part of the Israeli existence, while at the same time casting increasing doubt on the decision makers' wisdom" (Harel, 2013). Harel further quotes Nahum Barnea, a senior Israeli journalist for the *Yediot Aharonot*:

> The influence of the "Four Mothers" . . . accelerated processes that changed the attitude towards war and to the IDF within Israeli society. Falling in battle lost its legitimacy. . . . A civilian killed by a missile is presented as a personal tragedy: a soldier who is killed is presented as a national catastrophe.

A manifestation of the fact that uncontained parental anxiety over their sons' lives moves reciprocally into the sons' emotional state of mind can be found in the harsh words of a song lyric written by Erez Stark, who describes how a soldier son, thinking about death in the battle, does not cry over his own demise but over his sense of guilt towards his parents:

> If you're standing here above me,
> I guess I didn't keep my promise,
> Sorry, I really am, sorry,
> On my life I'm sorry . . .

The roles have been reversed: instead of the parents calming the son with "no harm will come to *you*", the son calms the parents with "no harm will come to *me*". Interestingly, the songwriter includes hurt from a woman and harm caused by a terrorist in the same sentence, as though pacifying the mother with the idea that the world she tried to build for her son, free from pain, threats, danger, and conflict, indeed exists. The cynicism in this song criticizes mothers sharply for raising their child this way.

The impact of parental interference and intervention on military functioning

Clearly it is not easy to be an Israeli youth, undergoing processes of maturation while readying for combat service, especially so in light of parental patterns shown in the interviews. However, despite mothers' wish to prevent their sons from becoming combatants and distance them from the image of the combat soldier, this is not the reality generally encountered: most soldiers are tough, determined, and highly motivated.

Kolonimus and Bar-Tal (2011) researched one hundred combat soldiers who, at the time of their recruitment, were imbued with positive expectations and displayed high motivation to enlist for the IDF, serve in elite combat units, and contribute to their country. They perceived serving in these units as the opportunity to develop and maximize their personal potential. There was also the halo of prestige around these units. The soldiers reported that the army assists the process of maturation and allows them to develop skills, perspectives, and values. Prior to recruitment, they had viewed violent action as a factor that promotes and confirms their masculinity. The pleasure they derive from strength and control is evident. Those who had completed their service felt that their exposure to war, injury, or death of mates had matured them. The army allowed them to grow up and develop deep friendships, independent capability, and a sense of meaningfulness, all of which they later implemented in civilian life.

Since the image of the combat soldier is one of hegemonic masculine identity in Israel, and since with his actual body he symbolizes the full connection between masculinity and nationality (Sasson-Levy, 2006), there is hardly any doubt why such intertwined motifs appear in statements made by soldiers when they describe their motivation for combat service.

It is evident that Ido and Ziv, whom I interviewed, the Nahal Brigade soldiers with whom Harel (2013) spoke, and soldiers interviewed by Yinon Mills (discussed below) are all "cast from the same mould". Together, their words show soldiers willing to give their lives, on condition that they know their actions are directed towards saving their country and family. From this perspective, the soldier of today hardly falls short of the mythological fighting-soldier hero of previous generations.

Tamir, interviewed by Harel (2013), described how, months prior to recruitment, he began working out three times a week. He was not sure whether he was suited to combat activity, but thinks he might be. He did not perceive of himself as spoilt and had no problem with discipline; he felt he could cope with tougher people. He knew that distancing from home would not be easy, but that if other people could do it, then he could too.

I am not familiar with Tamir's history, and nothing can be concluded about the source of his abilities from the few published interview sentences (Harel, 2013). However, we saw that his mother expressed the conflict she felt around his recruitment as a combat soldier through her contradictory statements: her anxiety over her sons from their moment of birth, and through her snooping, non-releasing behaviour. Tamir testified from the outset that "a home-front role is not an option in this household" and that joining the Nahal Brigade is perceived almost as a family project. Perhaps this is how the mother contained the conflict, including the burden of anxiety towards Tamir's life, thereby releasing him and allowing him to organize himself towards recruitment.

Ilay, aged eighteen and a half, also reflected these ideas when interviewed by Harel (2013). He is conscious of the existence of a dual motivator when enlisting for combat units: "There's the national aspect, to protect the country, and there's also the personal aspect. I'm taking it as a great experience for me."

Ido, whom I interviewed, also emphasized the aspect of responsibility towards the country. He explained that it wasn't that he wanted to fight, but to protect his country. "I don't want to do guard duty [in a settlement]. For that, there are security companies. I enlisted because there's an army, and my goal is to win the next war."

In an interview with Yinon Mills, from the *Yediot Aharonot* website,[18] Avihai described the moment that he felt his actions in Gaza were saving the home, when he discovered a shaft built for launching missiles and aimed at Israel:

> I think that the feeling of justice was so much in our emotions . . . Then we discovered a shaft, a missile launching shaft!!! . . . I think it was just about the only time that tears fell from my eyes. The thrill . . . the thrill . . . and not just me . . . I think most of the company, it makes your heart beat wildly. Because you go in, fight, you remember that you're protecting the State of Israel, and the people of Israel, and when you find a shaft at the precise angle . . . it's a chilling moment . . . I think that it's a moment that will stay with me from the war . . . we're actually saving people! This is us keeping guard over the State of Israel.

Support by commanders during war

In light of the effect of parental intervention on the authority and command of various military ranks, Ido's and Ziv's sense of this issue during the war was diametrically opposite, which sharpens understanding of the attitudes they were lacking when training. With confidence and satisfaction they talked about the commanders who, right before entering the war, had told them that they support them and will back them, whatever they think is the right thing to do. As Ido explained:

> "Suddenly you know that you're standing there, and everyone's got your back, and it's something that has to be done, and you're not the only one to understand that, everyone does. This perception significantly changed my attitude towards the soldiers and the soldiers' own attitudes."

I understood that initially he was deeply concerned that he could be judged for what he actually does in battle, and I asked him about it. Ido's response made me realize yet another issue that the protective parenting does not ready sons for: the dilemmas they face when needing to take action that opposes their moral values. The descriptions offered by Ido and Ziv demonstrate the complex emotional coping in which they found themselves and will probably need to cope with all their lives:

> "Yeah, because you do these things that you don't really accept. For example . . . Hamas fired really heavy anti-tank weapons which could hit you, from mosques! . . . To fire at mosques is not a simple decision to make . . . but when you have no other choice, you don't want to be sitting ducks, and you do things because they need to be done.
>
> Or for instance, in the tank . . . it was me that did the actual firing. And it's a really serious matter . . . most of the day what you're doing is scanning and thinking. And then, right after attacks where you fire and fire, you know that in some cases you've harmed people. And you've blown up houses because they're booby-trapped . . . and there's not much of them left. And you say: 'Someone was in there' but . . . it could be that I also just saved five people, because there were terrorists in there, and ten minutes later a team of five of our guys went in. So because of me, our guys didn't have to tackle them . . ."

Ziv described the importance of commanders' backing in such situations:

> "Listen, it doesn't matter what you're doing, if you have any doubt, first shoot and then ask questions. We'll back you up." It was good

> to hear that because until now, for instance, when I was on the Jenin front . . . you weren't allowed to do a thing. Someone can shoot at you, put his weapon down and his hands up, and you can't do a thing to him, nothing. In Gaza they supported everything you did, and it gave a much better feeling. You could protect yourself better."

Ido's and Ziv's descriptions hone in on the question of whether the young men can be better prepared for these complex emotional states. Perhaps, as David said (in chapter three), encountering the emotional complexity of this reality as parents of sons causes parents to ignore these issues; but ignoring them leaves the son-soldier to face these extremely complicated dilemmas alone.

The emotional significance of home-front backing during war

Ido and Ziv described the great relief and empowerment they felt, following weeks of tough fighting in Gaza, because of the emotional, moral, and material backing of the nation. This support was a determining factor in the soldiers' sense of strength and robustness and their willingness to fight, but also in their ability to leave the war with their psyches whole. It is moving to realize how critical this public backing is for them.

In my view, the intensity surfacing from their comments, and their enthusiasm, gratitude, and sense of tremendous relief, attest to the depth of distress they felt when retaliating to attacks in urban environments, knowing that civilians would inevitably be harmed; it also attests to their ability to contain the conflictual feelings engendered and begin talking and thinking about them.

The deep relief they spoke of derived not only from the stress of a young soldier finding himself in war situations, but from the fact that he enters the war bearing uncontained parental anxiety, lacking the paternal masculine guiding voice from the past, which is therefore not internalized and not available in the present. It may be the public voice, expressed in the clearest of terms and now encompassing a sense of responsibility towards the soldiers, that allowed them to connect to this vital function and feel themselves to be combat men ready for the tough mission ahead.

> "When you go into Gaza, you suddenly get that this is it, you understand why you're doing it, and you go in full force. . . . There was a lot of friction with Hamas. And you go in and start fighting, and it's all chaos.

> But the hard part really starts . . . once the first big attack is over, and suddenly you . . . switch from attack to the stage of protecting. *What I felt the strongest, and that kept me going there, was the support from the people.* You're constantly getting donations, huge packages of nibbles . . . *and you know it's all donated by people who really care."*

Ido described the abundance showered on them, particularly when they came out for a refresher break at the border:

> "Letters people wrote . . . pictures drawn by children, we'd tape them on . . . The whole thing was covered in pictures drawn by children: doodles, 'From Nursery school . . .', whatever its name was . . . all the kinds of things little kids do when they're told 'draw something for our soldiers'. And it really keeps you going.
>
> And every time you came out for a break, people made you a barbecue, brought you pizzas. They built field showers and brought them to where soldiers were . . . Crates on crates of donations. You understand that the people really care, that it's not a worthless thing. It's hard to digest. *In the end, that's what holds you up, that you know you're not out there alone and will cop criticism later.*
>
> A lot of people wrote their phone number on what they sent, and if we could, we phoned, 'Hello, I'm Ido, I'm in a tank, we've received your package, thanks so much'. *It makes us feel so good, it's amazing, really.* The whole country was with you!"

Brothers in arms: the bond of mutuality

Hanoch Yerushalmi (1997), who served as a military psychologist for one of the IDF's commando units, sheds light on another unconscious emotional dynamic aroused during military service. The experience of "brothers in arms" is central to the soldier during training in peacetime, but far more so during a war. As Yerushalmi explained, the main activity in commando units is training in survival techniques and destruction of the enemy. Daily activities and discussion therefore revolve around topics of life and death, which comprise the Israeli military reality on the one hand, and the world of phantasy on the other. To prepare themselves for a possible attack on their lives, soldiers frequently practise reactions in dangerous situations, the primary need being to learn to control fear.

Under such circumstances, the feeling of brotherhood becomes more meaningful: it is perceived as the potential for saving a life and readies the soldier for the moment he may need to sacrifice his life to save that of his "brother". Total devotion to the other, absence of self, and total dependency on "brothers" arouse primitive infantile wishes and phantasies, which recall the unconditional and boundless love for the mother. The development of brotherhood therefore arouses longing and a kind of fusion characteristic of the primal object, causing a sense of regression in the maturing young man who has just foregone finding the object of love within his family and is left with libidinal hunger (Yerushalmi, 1997).

These emotions become a central component in the boys' identities and accompany them throughout their lives. Although every primal relationship between infant and mother is one of fusion, it may be that in some circumstances, when the relationship with the mother did not undergo the necessary processes of separation and individuation, it intensifies the characteristics of the process described by Yerushalmi.

Ido and Ziv related to the component of mutual dependence and responsibility when it was felt as giving confidence, and also in cases where it did not and caused a sense of anxiety and lack of confidence.

Ido spoke of how, as he was preparing to leave Gaza, he heard that a soldier had been captured. In that instant, everything changed for him:

> "The second I heard there was a kidnap, you know that until it's over, I'm here. It doesn't matter how exhausted you are, I know I'm here. It's so annoying that he got captured, I want to leave, but there's no chance I'd do that until things are resolved."

I said: "That's a very weighty feeling of responsibility." Ido answered:

> "That's how it is towards everyone, it's more an identification with the responsibility, in my view. Identification is the understanding that it could be any of us, and that's how I'd want it to be. Only when they told us that the guy was dead, and they'd buried what could be buried, then it's possible to leave."

Ido and Ziv identified with the "Hannibal procedure": if soldiers see a soldier being captured, they should try to shoot the captors, and if there's no choice, then the captured soldier. Ido said:

> "That's what has to be done. And I know that if I was the captured soldier, I'd also want them to do that."

Ziv added:

> "You know that that's how it's got to be, and it's the best thing because you know that if you do everything to prevent that kidnap, it'll cause a lot less kidnapping. I believe that even if I'd gotten to

> that state . . . that they'd kill me, it's what has to be done . . . it's so much bigger than you, and it's not meant to affect your calculations."

Ziv explained that if the enemy succeed in capturing once, they will attempt it again: today it could be him, tomorrow someone else. Both soldiers described their distress when their mates did not function according to this procedure.

The experience of gratification and excitement over the ability to rely absolutely on the other forces is emphasized in Ziv's remarks about being called into action to blow up numerous tunnels. Receiving permission to assist strengthened their feeling of being effective, reliable soldiers. When Ziv described the protective gear he wore, I realized that not all parts of his body were covered; I asked: "Were you afraid?" He answered:

> "It's scary, but it's not what protects me. What protects you are the people . . . when that tank suddenly turns up with its tremendous firing force, and technology, and people you can rely on."

Zev Shweidel, a mental evaluation officer in the war, was moved by the levels of support, love, and mutuality he met among the injured soldiers:

> "In my role as a reservist . . . I came across incredible pain of a kind I'd never been exposed to in my life. But in the same breath, I saw the pinnacles of love, support, compassion, and mutuality. These, you also don't see every day.
>
> I remember, for example, when I was called into the casualty ward by a soldier demanding to urgently see the mental evaluation officer. I rushed over, readying myself for a hysterical attack along the lines of 'I'm injured, I want to go home, I want my mother . . .' Instead, the blond soldier aged twenty said that he was only lightly injured, the shell shock he'd suffered was brief, and . . . he asked me to write that he's okay because he wants to go back to the fighting right away . . . After all, I'm the mental evaluation officer, and I'm there to help him not be psychologically stressed. And that's what would calm his stress . . ."

The "peacetime self" versus the "wartime self"

In 1948 there was no acknowledgment of psychic damage; the concept that there could be injury even when the physical body was not injured simply did not exist at the time (Levi, Witztum, Granek, & Kotler, 1989).[19] Psychological health researchers have dedicated abundant resources to exploring the phenomenon of "post-traumatic stress disorder"—a term that replaces Freud's "war neurosis". A good deal of professional attention has been devoted to defining those considered as having mental injuries from war, but there has been very little focus on understanding what occurs in the soldier's psyche—whether he himself fought, lost friends, or served during the war in a supportive role and was not diagnosed as a casualty.

Freud (1915c) explained that in wartime, as a result of the effect of danger to a soldier's life, a new, brave self is formed—a "wartime self"—that protects against danger. The "old self of peacetime" realizes that the new self endangers its existence, and conflict is thereby aroused. Freud noted that the ground that nurtures war neurosis is a People's Army, not a mercenary military. The wartime self remains embedded in the soldier even after discharge and surfaces in him as automatically as a serving soldier's response to the command "At attention" (Freud, 1914).

Ido described the sudden change of perception—"It happens in an instant"—occurring in himself and his mates in the unit on crossing the border into Gaza. "It becomes clear", he said, "that if you act normal, you won't survive . . . It's the clearest instinct of survival."

> "At the most basic level, you understand that all the training, all the exercises . . . this is the time to implement them. Then the routine becomes one of war . . . and you just know you're doing what has to be done, because there's no other way. You can't just leave the tank post now, because if that post isn't there, people will get killed. It makes no difference if you've slept or not, had time to eat, if something hurts . . . You do it, because . . . it needs to be done."

In actuality, this involves adjustment to a military environment to which the Israeli male may find himself returning annually as part of reserve duty, or when called up due to war. In both cases, the Israeli male will be required to switch between the two environments, each time activating a different kind of personality organization.

In *The Naked and the Dead* (1948), Norman Mailer writes about how putting on a helmet and flak jacket and carrying a few grenades and a weapon gives a sense of being bound with a tourniquet on both shoulders, and chest and limbs feel numbed. Perhaps this is the source of strength that Ido, Ziv, and their compatriots found to help them withstand the difficult conditions.

I asked whether they were afraid. Ido said:

> "You don't have time to be scared there. You're sharp, you understand the danger, but it isn't frightening. It's not like standing on the edge of a cliff and being scared.
>
> It's a different focus of your personality. . . . And people behave differently from usual. I have this really close friend, a fantastic commander, but . . . it was really, really hard for me with him, because under pressure he didn't function. It's tough for everyone, no matter what you're doing . . . I sit in the gunner's spot, with my legs folded under the seat, and I can't move left or right. The driver sits in a hermetically sealed cubicle. And his whole view of the world is the small periscope in front of his eyes. And that's how it is, for a day or more.
>
> Your legs go numb, your arms go numb, and it's really really uncomfortable. But if it were comfortable, you'd fall asleep. . . . after twenty-four hours sitting in the driver's cubicle, you're all alone, you don't see anyone. You have internal communication, but you're sitting there alone . . . it's really tough . . ."

Freud noted in a letter to Dr Frederik van Eeden regarding the impact of war that psychoanalysis had learned that the primitive, wild, evil drives of humanity have not disappeared but continue to exist, despite being in a repressed unconscious mode that awaits the opportunity to become active again (as cited in Jones, 1957). During military combat, the soldier may encounter in his psyche these emotional extremes that he may never have had to face in times of peace.

Sexual drives

When a flooding of stimuli occurs, the psychic system is pressured, regulatory defences loosen, and the intensity of sexual drive increases. During the course of commando training, *aggressive drives fuse with sexual drives* and create powerful motivational drives that boost soldiers' motivation and the strength to withstand the tough physical training. However, this may come with an emotional price.

Relieving these intertwined aggressive and sexual drives can be seen in poems composed by the soldiers themselves, replete with aggressive sexual content towards women. Milo (2012) studied 663 such poems composed between 1940 and 2008 and found that, despite the improved status of women in Israeli society throughout these seven decades, the soldiers' poems and songs show no change: the masculine model of the warrior is still the dominant one.

The integration of women into commando activities led to a radicalization of the female image in soldiers' songs, as in one song from the Givati Brigade. The commander referred to here carries the feminine gender identifier in the original Hebrew:

> Aaaah, we've raped another commander/we've raped the bitch/she went and complained/complained to the police/and the unit's being investigated/and to the unit, absentee/to the unit, deserters/to the unit light drugs/to the unit heavy drugs/and all of me all of me's aggravated/the heart's shaking with aggro.

This song creates a climate in which sex and violence are bound into each other as a comprehensible—though not legitimate—response by the vengeful fighter who is above the law. It is a social atmosphere in which the threat of sexual aggression is perceived as legitimate within the masculine military discourse. This phenomenon also manifests in giving female names to the hills where training takes place, exercises typically involving "charging Hamotal" and "conquering Mira", creating an atmosphere that impacts the attitude in the base.

The commando identifies strongly with his weapon, his tool of control: to him the feminine is therefore a target of conquest. Scorn is also directed towards the non-combatant "jobnik" soldier.

Slavin and Kriegman (1992, cited in Yerushalmi, 1997) view the reappearance of repressed drives, and the "self–other" relationship patterns, as processes needed for adaptation to the new environment and its new conditions in the adult world, which occurs simultaneously with negotiation with that environment. The encounter with this environment allows the maturing soldier to accept new concepts relative to his personality, since the concept is broader than that which he experienced within his family.

The dynamic of the reappearing sexual drives typical of the sexual maturity stage, together with the oedipal competition, become powerful and therefore more difficult to regulate in the military environment. The internalization of this renewed oedipal resolution does not provide life-tools for subsequent functioning in the civilian environment, which places the young Israeli in a unique and complicated conflict.

It is therefore no small wonder that these songs remain within the closed forum of male soldiers, unknown by the public. Soldiers' songs sung by the public show the opposite picture: a longing for the girlfriend at home or a plea to her not to cry over her dying soldier.

Perhaps a kind of separation has come about in the soldier's psyche between the instinctual libidinal function and the value-based function (of the superego), where the soldiers' songs show the freedom to talk of what is denied and not openly spoken about. The issue of the emotional significance of the process experienced by these young men and of ourselves as a society needs further study.

Aggressive/destructive drives

Theodor Nadelson (2005), a psychiatrist and psychoanalyst who worked with soldiers who had served in Vietnam, described the emotional process of the soldier during battle and after discharge. The first issue Nadelson needed to handle was the encounter between the soldier and his extreme destructive aggression. As one soldier told him about how he felt about fighting, "I'm afraid I enjoyed it"—adding, in a despairing tone: "What the heck is wrong with me?" Nadelson related how the soldiers discovered that social restraints from prior to the war disappeared in the war itself. They adopted the war, felt ready for it, and even operated from murderous fury. Their identity before this experience was nothing like their post-experience identity. The post-experience soldiers experienced gratification from destruction—the opposite of civilization.

Following from Nadelson, war can be seen as a modern induction ceremony, challenging its participants with the risk of death.

Freud explained that our unconscious is inaccessible to the image of the self's death, craving murder relative to the stranger and ambivalence relative to the beloved. War peels layers of later acculturation off us and discloses the primal human within. According to Freud (1915c), war coerces us into being heroes again, of a type that does not believe in the possibility of death relative to ourselves; war colours the foreigner as an enemy whose death must be longed for if not exacted; war instructs us to ignore the death of our loved ones.

In everyday life, Ido is a sensitive young man who plays music and sings. He devoted one year prior to recruitment to expanding his study of philosophy and general knowledge, while contributing to society. His words demonstrate the change from peacetime self to wartime self, according to Freud's (1915c) concept:

> "I had no problem with killing when I had to. I have no regrets, no pressures. Even when you shoot at people, you don't feel you're killing a person . . . And that's because there's not even one second of doubt. Because it's either him or . . . not necessarily just

me, because in the tank we were protected, but it could be my mates. Either they'll continue their shooting, or they'll be afraid to approach, that kind of thing."

It was impossible to ignore the excitement accompanying Ido's descriptions. However, it is worth noting that Ido's description is based on negation: "I had *no* problem with killing . . . I have *no* regrets . . . you *don't* feel you're killing". As discussed in chapter one, the purpose of negation is to filter emotional content from the conscious that is too harsh to contain by expressing the content via the negative (Freud, 1925). Like any soldier, it appears that Ido was indeed forced to experience his aggressive parts at their fullest force and cope with the pleasure he felt while experiencing them.

Prior to a battle, there is often enthusiasm for it to start—as voiced by Ariel, a soldier in compulsory service, who in an interview with Yinon Mills described how the weeks of waiting near the Gaza border felt:

> Everyone wanted to go in, bottom line. They were going nuts. I personally have been preparing for three years for this moment . . . and when we went in, we were supercharged, everyone slapping each other on the back, "I love you, bro . . . C'mon, let's go in . . . Headbutt them . . ." There was this serious atmosphere.

Yerushalmi (2008) offers an explanation for this longing to go into battle: for soldiers at war, the anxiety and phantasy over what will happen is a realistic nightmare, and they long to see the battle begin in order to be rid of the terrible anxiety building up.

Ziv and Ido described the war in factual terms and in fine detail—for example, Ido's remarks on active duty at problem locations, referred to with the regular war terminology of a "front":

> "When I was posted to a front in Israel, at the time some of our training seemed unnecessary. But once I got into Gaza . . . everything changed crazily . . . in war, it's a whole different world.
>
> Suddenly you're looking at some house and you see there are lights in there. And you ask for permission to shoot. You say you've identified someone, probably a terrorist. And you see that people are relying on you, they're relying completely, you're the one who's protecting . . ."

Ido and Ziv spoke for some two hours, almost without a break. It was evident that their detailing of the war's development allowed both of them a chance for emotional processing, which they later said they so badly needed, and they continued that conversation between them for a long time afterwards.

Frustration over stopping the war

In light of the surging sexuality, the frustration felt by Ziv over the cessation of Operation Protective Edge before fully realizing the ability to fight is natural:

> "Because they related to the whole thing as a specific campaign just to blow up all the tunnels, rather than totally wipe out the Hamas forces, it felt like we were being held back. For example, . . . terrorists shot at the house next to us with guns . . . and started running into Gaza. We were taught so far that every time they take a go at you, it's a signal for direct encounter, until the terrorist is taken out. And suddenly they didn't want us to go all the way into Gaza."

Attitudes towards death

Since commando service in Israel represents anxiety over the death of the soldier-son, as we have seen, the attitude towards death is woven like a thread through a soldier's life and constitutes the most important component impacting his development and identity.

During World War I, Freud (1915c) studied attitudes towards death. He noted how, despite an individual's acknowledgment of the fact that eventually we all die, in actuality it is harder for us to imagine our own death: in other words, at the unconscious level, each of us is convinced of our own immortality, and therefore we try to ignore the existence of death and conceal it from our lives. Freud explains that this defence collapses with the death of someone close to us; then something inside us dies too, and together with that person we bury our hopes, expectations, and pleasures, refusing any alternative to them. This approach to death has significant influence on us and may prevent us from living life courageously. When we no longer dare to take risks, life becomes impoverished, a wrapper with no content.

In Israel, the encounter with death of family and friends in various wars, and certainly through unconscious intergenerational baggage, caused a sense of apprehension, to the extent that commanders' freedom to appropriately train their soldiers was harmed.

Freud further explained that throughout human development, additional approaches to death have developed: thoughts on the souls of the dead, belief in the immortality of the soul, and consciousness of guilt that gave birth to the first moral commands, of which the most significant is "You shall not murder". Gradually, explains Freud, this reaction also spread relative to unloved foreigners and finally applied also to enemies. Nevertheless, the victorious fighter will return home joyfully to his family, unchecked and undisturbed by thoughts of those he has killed (Freud, 1915c).

The encounter between soldiers and death includes the possibility of their own death, the killing of the enemy, seeing enemy corpses, and witnessing or coping with the death of fellow soldiers and friends.

Ariel and Avihai, interviewed by Yinon Mills, related to the moment that they realized their lives were in danger. Their remarks demonstrate how the mechanism described by Freud makes it harder to accept the possibility of our own death.

Ariel spoke first, describing how they scouted the area and actually put their heads outside the tank. They heard shots, but he didn't connect this with the idea that someone was shooting at him. It was only when his commander shouted, "We're being shot at! Get inside!" that he realized that "they want to kill us! Suddenly the penny dropped: someone's trying to kill me! He described the chilling feeling in that first instant of being shot at and how his hands began to shake.

Ariel took in another aspect of death when a wounded terrorist attempted to continue fighting, and one of the commanders shot him. Despite the terrorist's lower body being trapped under the ruins, he was trying to crawl out holding his weapon. "It was a scary image", Ariel said, and continued:

> One of the commanders cocked his gun and shot. So when we got there, we saw the guy, smashed on the floor, all covered in blood. Like, I don't know . . . it's tough, it's . . . damn . . . Dunno . . . what have we come to??? Damn, it's like really shitty . . . it's a disgusting thing.

He added that he had never before seen a person in that state, but he had to look because "in the end that's what has to be done, because it's either him or us, so there's no choice, you have to look".

When the situation involves an entire country under attack, there is no doubt that war becomes a necessity, as noted by Winnicott (1940) when he referred to World War II and his very pragmatic stance that the war is in order to exist: the fight, he explained, is simply because we don't want to be destroyed or subjugated, and there's nothing extraordinary about that. His pragmatism went further: victory must be a victory of superiority in war; if by contrast an artificial peace is made prior to one side proving their military superiority beyond all doubt, the old problems of blame for the war will resurface, and the peace we wish for will again fail.

Ido, with considered honest clarity, said that, by definition, it's forbidden for a kidnap to happen.

> "There just cannot be such a thing as you're being kidnapped, because the price of a kidnapping is much more significant than a killing. And it sounds terrible, but that's how it is."

I found myself wondering out loud: "What amazes me is that you talk straightforwardly from a place of understanding and acceptance that you're willing to die in order to protect others, so there won't be an even harsher price." Ziv responded:

> "I believe everyone needs to think that way. If everyone thinks that way, it closes the gaps—that way no one gets hurt . . . If everyone's protecting himself, there'll be loads of small spots of protection, but if everyone's protecting others, it creates a much bigger field, stronger, and no one can get hurt."

At that point I asked: "And are you trained to think this way, or is this a personal conclusion?" Ido answered first: "We're taught that, but, bottom line, you also need to absorb it for yourself." Ziv added: "You have to believe in it."

Their words were hard for me to acknowledge. I found it difficult to see how they could hold such stances, even when no longer in war situations, despite being the "children raised on cream", pampered, identifying with values of life and pleasure. I set a tougher base when I turned to Ido and asked how he got to that moment when he could say, "Me, a guy who loves life, I am willing to die, and my heart is in it".

Ido thought quietly, concentrating, as though seeking inside his psyche for an answer. His response left me open-mouthed and moved:

> *"It's from my love of life. If you love life, it's no problem. If you love only your own life, it's a lot harder.* It means looking a bit beyond yourself. Because if you look only at yourself, the *moment* your guard's down you'll get hurt, and so will everyone else around you. But if you know that when his guard's down you're looking out for him, and when your guard's down he's looking out for you, this understanding is, bottom line, what keeps you strong.

If you love life, you don't watch out only for your own life, you watch out for the lives of everyone around you. It's like a spreading circle. Whoever's around you, whatever you can contain. If you can contain everyone around you, then you're also part of that, and your life is part of the totality, of everything."

These responses echo again the different emotional dynamics Freud (1915c) identified that distance consciousness of death during war. Freud notes that war must sweep away the accepted approach towards death. It can no longer be denied: people truly die—nor is it just one death, but a large number. Moreover, their deaths are no longer subject to coincidence; in fact, if even one bullet hits one person, almost certainly a second bullet will hit someone else. The false impression over chance death thus ends, and life becomes interesting again, since it has been reimbued with content. Freud suggests that it might have been better to give a little more emphasis to the position of the unconscious, to death, which we repress so devotedly. He then quotes (in Latin) an old adage, "If you want peace, prepare for war", but he twists it slightly to, "If you would endure life, be prepared for death".

During Operation Protective Edge, and for several weeks after it ended, a drama workshop was held for soldiers in the framework of the Kibbutz College.[20] On the final evening, the group presented theatrical skits that they had created, including a piece written by one of the group, Nitai Schmeltzer, that demonstrates coping with the experience of death.

The action takes place in an apartment in Gaza. Three soldiers, Yohai, Eden, and Tom, wake up and are singing as they getting organized. It is a song in which the phrase "eternal tranquillity", a euphemism for death, appears repeatedly. They wonder if the ceasefire will hold, doubting it will. In the discussion they find it difficult to contain their experiences, such as indecisiveness on the part of commanders. To Yohai's remark that he wants to "get into the war already", that he'll "go all the way to the sea, whatever's needed, that's the only way there'll be quiet", Eden responds cynically: "Yohai, calm down, you forget you're in a risk group." Yohai questions what he means.

Eden: "Death doesn't just take people randomly. It chooses them with a tweezer. For instance, you, Yohai, you're getting married in a month, a classic death . . ."

Then he begins to mouth phrases as though quoting from obituaries for each of them in newspapers after their deaths.

The skit, replete with bitterly cynical remarks, looks death in the eye and slowly moves to acceptance of it. The Angel of Death enters the room in a black cloak, its face whitened. Eden and Yohai befriend Death, offer it food, and talk with it. Tom gives Death a physical domain between Nir Oz, a kibbutz in which terror tunnels were found, and Khan Younis, a Gazan town just inside the border, saying to them:

> Tom: "Hey, what are you talking with it for? That garbage is wandering about for a week already between Nir Oz and Khan Younis, doing anything it wants, taking who it wants, finishing people's lives up."

> Death: "Hullo! It's not like how you say it is. All in all, I'm just fulfilling my orders . . . I don't really choose . . ."

Death justifies its actions by claiming it is simply fulfilling its role, just as they fulfil theirs. With this sentence, Nitai is perhaps trying to digest the fact that, in war, he also caused the death of others, which carries with it emotional difficulty.

> Death (standing up): "D'you think it's easy to be me? There isn't a single person who doesn't judge me, everyone curses me . . . thinks I'm some kind of evil bastard who does what he wants without taking anyone into consideration. No one thinks about me, the things I need to see, the experiences I undergo . . . no one says to me, 'Good for you, Death, that's good work you're doing', or 'Nice job, Death. Why not take off early today . . .'"
>
> Tom: "What do you want? That we'll pass before you one at a time and kiss your feet?!"
>
> Death: "No. But I expect you to give me the minimum respect I deserve and realize that, like with every job, there are constraints, there are orders, and the mission must be fulfilled!"

The skit ends with the three soldiers organizing themselves, getting geared up, checking all kinds of things in preparation. At the same time, Death, on the other side of the stage, stands up and is buzzed on the radio.

> Death: "This is Death. Over." (*Listens.*) "Repeat." (*Listens.*) "All three?" (*Listens.*) "Over and out." (*Sits down heavily.*)
>
> Eden (*approaches Death*): "C'mon Death, you coming? In a minute we need to quit this building."

Death does not react. Eden looks at Yohai and Tom, who are also approaching.

Yohai: "What's up, Death? Why're you so bummed out?"

Death (*whispering*): "I got this command."

Eden: "Okay. We did too. What are you so emotional about, we're all pros here."

Death (*looking at them*): "I got an order."

There is silence. Death stands slowly.

Tom: "And it's . . . final?"

Death: "Yeah."

Through humour, the soldiers are able to touch on the death they cause to civilians, and the death that is waiting in ambush for them. They accept the fact that, on the one hand, they are fulfilling orders and taking responsibility and, on the other, after acknowledging the various functions they fill in this tough war, they are able to return from their leave to the battlefield.

The moral stance

Unlike the description Freud (1915c) offered for the emotional state of the soldier returning from battle lacking any care for the fate of the enemy and even celebrating that enemy's death, the Israeli soldiers presented here experienced feelings of pain when exposed to the enemy's humanity and through identification with the destruction caused to the Gazans despite the need for their actions. Ariel spoke of having to overcome these sensations in order to carry on:

> "Our mission was to get the homes, search for tunnels, search for weapons, search for observation posts. I remember seeing a crib positioned in this really weird angle . . . and mattresses all arranged on one side, for seven kids. And you know that because someone used this house as an observation post, they won't have a house anymore. Seven kids, and this is their house. As a father, I feel just how much a house is a home. They're important, these four walls, roof, kitchen, bathroom, and all of that will stop existing . . . I need . . . I felt that I need to take hold of myself . . . and it's clear to me that because I have two kids, it was so strong . . . It's a painful feeling, but that's what needs to be done."

Dr Ben Haroush, who also fought in Gaza and participated in the same interview, described in an emotionally distanced manner how, even during warfare, his moral codes remained very clear to him:

> "We reached the first line of houses, and in one they shot into a cupboard that looked suspicious. Some guy fell out unarmed, so we quickly gave him first aid and morphine. One of the soldiers said, 'Why are you giving him morphine, maybe he's a terrorist' (which in fact he was), but he was unarmed. I also said, 'When a person's wounded and doesn't constitute a threat and isn't fighting, then he needs to get treatment, like anybody else.' That's my education from home, and from medical college."

When asked if he would treat someone even if he knew that person had shot a missile at his house and endangered his family, he agreed it was a dilemma, but he would nevertheless help him: "It's not my position to make decisions about who to judge, punish and so on."

The ability to see the enemy as human manifests when the interviewer asked how Gaza looked. All three interviewees were able to note its beauty and vitality before the war, and the destruction in the wake of war. Ariel said that he could see it had been really lovely before they went in. Avihai added that "it's really pretty, they have these courtyards with grass and cool landscaped parks". Ariel remarked that nothing much remained alive afterwards. The destruction was pretty complete.

When Ariel was asked whether any of his views had changed due to the war, those deriving from his internalized experiences were evident. He said that he used to be fiercely right wing but now felt unsure about how to define himself, "because all this situation of war is like poison. People die on us, people die on them too. It's not important how many of us or them—people simply die. I think about my country in twenty years . . . I don't want this to carry on". Avihai added that he is "tired of living by the sword". "But I don't have any choice. It's a pretty frustrating feeling."

No doubt even now it is still too early to write about the war and its soldiers. As I noted earlier, I suspect I am using writing and rationalization as a defence mechanism, in an effort to create a space for reflection on developing the emotional and cognitive ability that will allow observing, containing, and symbolizing occurrences beyond the survival reactions when under conditions of attack.

Conclusions

Having reviewed several of the milestones of the Israeli military and, correspondingly, several of the characteristics comprising the identity of the Israeli soldier, it becomes possible to identify a similarity developing in both. In general, it can be said that the realistic danger of extermination with which the young State of Israel, and its newly established army, was threatened reconstructed the traumas of the people in the Holocaust—traumas so horrific that they could not be emotionally processed and internalized. This proximity of events created an emotional dynamic of splitting between the despairing, helpless victim attitude and the messianic, omnipotent, miraculous and heroic attitude that pacifies the oppositional victimhood. The victories of the War of Independence, the Sinai War, and the Six Day War reinforced the sense of miraculous omnipotence, with opposing voices excluded, and became part of the soldier's and military's identity. In the Yom Kippur War, however, the perception of "victim or omnipotent" still held, but the lack of preparedness of the IDF and other negative events during the war allowed the "other side of the coin" to surface: the sense of victimhood and despair.

An essential change to this split stance may be evident from the integration of various circumstances and factors: the move from a generation of Holocaust survivors experiencing incursions from neighbouring Arab countries to a generation born in Israel, in a young yet independent country with a unique identity; the military's need to conduct warfare in populated areas, which brought soldiers into direct contact with enemy civilian populations; and retaliation against terror attacks on the Israeli civilian population—the intifadas, the Lebanon wars, and the wars in Gaza. The split developed into an integrative one that allows acknowledging situations that mix bravery and resourcefulness with fear and helplessness; awareness of the justness of military action with the ability to acknowledge the pain and harm suffered by the enemy; and observation and reflection on the overall situation, rather than just seeing things from the Israeli perspective.

If the significance of this process is not understood, expressions relating to the pain of the other, or feelings that express something other than omnipotence, may be taken as indicating social and personal disintegration rather than stages needed for maturation that actually indicate psychic cohesion and personality integration. This insight is confronted by comments such as those of Oz Almog:[21]

> Up until the Yom Kippur War the State of Israel was a "society of vision" directed at national goals. . . . Over time, it lost its innocence and its tribal solidarity, and became more critical, quarrelsome, and egocentric. This is a dramatic change, in Israeli terms, where most Israelis are conscious of its occurrence, but simultaneously suppress

> its far-reaching significance. We came to the land to build and be built by it. But it is doubtful whether the image of the yuppie were part of the plans of the founding generation.

The understanding reached in this chapter is consistent with that of Shalvi (2016): that the image of the Israeli soldier underwent a change from being unidimensional, typified by heroism, to being multidimensional, which, in addition to characteristics of commando masculinity, allowed it to continue being attached to its softer layers.

An expression of this understanding can be found in the visual media. Over the first two decades of Israel's existence, the figure of the soldier was used in advertising: the very fact of a soldier recommending any item promoted its sale among the admiring public. From the 1970s, however, the use of military symbols in product advertising decreased in general, and emphasis was placed on a personal approach based on identification and caring concern. The soldier was presented as a young person fulfilling his duty but not necessarily always enjoying it (Rubin-Sagi, 1998).

The photographer Adi Ness identifies the Israeli soldier at the time of Israel's establishment as the hero, cast in the strong, contrasting Israeli light, a mythical spirit pervading the photographs. After the Yom Kippur War, the soldier has a more human aura, the sloppy reservist, with a beer belly, in ashen tones. Then, in his 2008 series of photographs, the soldiers are always in "a time that is no time, and a place that is no medium . . . and this soldier says: 'I'm everyman, every citizen, I'm not necessarily Israeli, and I don't even have the IDF logo on my shirt.'"[22] His photographs of Israeli soldiers from the War of Independence and the Six Day War reflect the end of the euphoric Zionist phase and the disintegration of the myth of the masculine soldier, inserting instead homoerotic elements. Zilberstein (2013), who reviewed the image of the soldier in theatre and film, also concluded that initially the image is whole but subjugated to its heroic role or presented as components of a national narrative and message. In the second stage, doubt appears, and the figure is vulnerable at the personal, social, historical, and theatrical levels, to the point of the absurd and pathological. The third stage contains the shattering and refutation of the meaning of war, the legendary figure, and the myth of soldiers, who also appear as marionettes destined for extinction or as robots without ideology. The films Zilberstein discusses emphasize the soldier's body, the presence of death, and the significance of time. It is especially worth noting that the image of the dead soldier is a common one in Israeli films.

When Melanie Klein (1946) predicated the existence of two emotional attitudes—splitting, an experience of black and white, and the integrative position, in which good and bad function interchangeably—she stressed that these are two emotional positions that the individual naturally moves between. There should be no expectation, therefore, that we, as a society, family, or individual, should be able to preserve the integrative position permanently. Rather, we should be conscious of it, identify the situations in which our experiences are split, are right and wrong, hero and victim, and try to return to the ability for an integrative experience that identifies in the individual, family, and society that range of changing emotions from one state to the other. Reasonably, the emotional stance in a state of war would be typified by the split characteristics described above. However, in order to understand what happens in the psyche of post-war soldiers when they return to normal civilian and family life, further research is essential.

Notes

1. It is impossible in one chapter to do justice to such a broad topic. In-depth study would require, for example, relating to the values of and emotional processes experienced by soldiers in compulsory service compared to reserves, those in different types of military corps, and the different modes and nature of combat, etc. Separate study should be made relative to different populations such as Israeli-born versus new immigrants, non-Jewish populations, the religious sector, etc. All this can be doubled when relating separately to women in the military.

2. The president of Israel, Reuven Rivlin, is a member of such a family, for example.

3. The following chain of events was written freely with references from Wikipedia and other research materials for factual verification.

4. Wikipedia: "Lessons of the Lebanon War", 25 August 2014.

5. The survey was conducted by the Public Opinion Research Institute; 378 overseas volunteers were interviewed, primarily young single men from English-speaking countries. The survey was conducted again on Israel's 66th Independence Day. The survey is available (in Hebrew) at www.idi.org.il/media/3159358/mahal_survey.pdf

6. A Romanian term imported into the Hebrew language referring to insider contacts.

7. This quote comes from an article (in Hebrew) on the official IDF site on 19 August 2014 (http://mazi.idf.il/4634-5243-HE/IGF.aspx). Israeli history and its development is indeed presented to currently serving soldiers as part of their identity and battle heritage.

8. *Ha'aretz*, 14 May 2008.

9. Moshe Dayan commanded the Etzioni Brigade in 1948 and was Minister of

Defence in 1967; Ariel Sharon commanded a platoon in the Alexandroni Brigade in 1948 and Battalion 38 in 1967; Motti Hod participated in the Velveta Campaign in 1948 smuggling Spitfires from Czechoslovakia to Israel, and commanded the Israel Air Force in 1967; Yitzhak Rabin fought in the Palmach in 1948 and was Chief of Staff in 1967.

10. Zev Schiff, *Ha'aretz*, 30 April 1968 (cited in Gan, 2009).

11. Retrieved from the Monosson Archive: www.ynet.co.il/articles/0,7340,L-3724195,00.html

12. Ilana Dayan, leading the *Uvdah* (Hebrew: Fact) television programme, 3 April 2008.

13. From the Latin *simulare*, "similarity", "parallel".

14. *Bamakhaneh* is the official IDF weekly journal, presenting articles from the soldiers' lives.

15. Which Klein called "depressive".

16. I feel it worthwhile to emphasize yet again that in-depth psychoanalytic research is needed to study these processes in our psyches.

17. A sizeable number of these standards were not implemented due to excessive parental intervention until the lessons from numerous and horrifying accidents were learned. Nonetheless, Ziv's words raise a relevant question on this issue.

18. Interview [in Hebrew] transcribed from a YouTube clip on "Tzuk Eitan": http://news.nana10.co.il/Article/?ArticleID=1077330.

19. Meir Pa'il, a historian who fought in the War of Independence and held senior command roles, was involved in the education of commandos and considered shell-shock to be somewhere between cowardice and "hysterical reaction". Research conducted in 1989 into individuals suffering from combat reactions from the past revealed that no documentation existed on the history of treating, or relating to, shock reactions in the IDF. As with other military forces, the "tradition" continued of forgetting or repressing the knowledge and lessons on this topic between one war and the next, and each generation pays the price for "reinventing the wheel" (Levi et al., 1989).

20. The Drama Workshop for Soldiers, under the auspices of the Kibbutz College, led by musician Boaz Debi and Yaron Edelstein.

21. Available at: www.peopleil.org/details.aspx?itemID=7730

22. https://www.youtube.com/watch?v=KSqJuQ4wcsA

CHAPTER EIGHT

After discharge: withdrawal into travel, mysticism, and blunting of the senses

Discharge from military service[1] brings the young Israeli, who has served as a commando dealing with challenging emotional processes, face to face with the expectation of integrating into Israeli society as a productive adult with an emotion-regulating masculine identity with its uniquely Israeli civilian facets. However, the discharged soldier is also expected to remain connected with those commando parts of his personality in order to have an integrated personality/self, and also because he may be drafted for reserve duty once a year. Without doubt, in-depth research is needed into this difficult transition, implementing psychoanalytic tools (PQRM; Mann-Shalvi, 2007b), together with a focus on concealed and revealed psychic layers in order to evaluate the emotional processes undergone by the young Israeli on his way from protected infancy to commando, and from commando to civilian.

Examination of the emotional processes experienced by the young Israeli who served in a combat role during this limbo stage of his life revealed three possible sources of emotional distress encountered in the process of consolidating his masculine identity after military service:

1. Unprocessed traumatic experiences from the military service period.
2. Interrupted maturation-development continuity.
3. Guilt and compensation as components in the structure of the parent–son relationship.

When these processes are latent, their influence is frequently erroneously attributed to irrelevant causes.

Unprocessed traumatic experiences from the military service period

Ziv, who was discharged two weeks before we met, just days after he had fought in Gaza, felt that all the responsibility for his life had fallen on his shoulders at once, without time to get used to it. He was pressured at first, feeling that he couldn't do anything well, and became depressed sometimes. When people said, "Hey, calm down, bro', it's just two weeks", he replied, "What, two weeks . . . I haven't managed to do a thing":

> "When you're in the army you're part of this huge strong organization, with a solid feeling of belonging. And in this war you felt you not only belonged to your unit but also to your people. It's really being a part of a tapestry. As strange as that sounds, in some way it's ideal because you bring yourself to your maximum capability, and you're also contained and held to the maximum. So suddenly in one go you're ejected from all that—it really feels like being ejected into space."

The difficulty in transitioning from commando life to civilian life may manifest in travel in the form of backpacking or trekking, whether as a kind of moratorium before shouldering other responsibilities or as escapism, a rejection of life. Each year, some fifty thousand discharged Israeli soldiers travel overseas for what has become known as "the great trek", usually to cheaper destinations in Asia or the Americas (Noy, 2007). A few make it all the way to Australia and New Zealand. The use of drugs, particularly cannabis-related products, is considered normal and acceptable among these young adults (Boni, 2012).

An illusion exists in Israeli society that when these discharged soldiers return from "their great trek", all their life experiences so far will disappear in some wondrous way—both having been overprotected and/or pampered children and the life-shaking experiences they faced in the army. The assumption is that they will now continue their proper development as functioning men—as though their lives were one continuum and combat service is just a natural stage within it (Mann-Shalvi, 2007b).

Indeed, most of the backpackers state that they went for the purpose of a change, and to "clean out our heads", even if they were not sure just what the change is. The trek, usually undertaken with others, is a kind of entry ticket into that club of young people seeking their desired identity. This may be why the phenomenon has collective normative, if not downright conformational, traits. In fact, Israeli society virtually expects a combat soldier to go trekking after being discharged; if he doesn't go, he feels he must justify his decision (Noy, 2007).

What drives young Israelis to trek is a question that preoccupied the musicians Yinon bar Shira and Becca Bar, who produced a rock musical entitled *Trip*.[2] Yinon wrote the musical after a close friend was killed on just such a post-discharge trek. The musical describes four young guys trekking in a dangerous jungle: three of them take hallucinatory drugs and return to repressed traumatic moments of their military service that they had hoped would remain in the depths of their psyches. Slowly the situation becomes increasingly dangerous, with no rescue mission for memories, and their memories begin to endanger even their "trekking lives".

In light of the lack of social discourse on this topic and of a framework to assist in coping, this difficult stage of transition from military to civilian life is largely ignored in Israeli society. Studies that have explored this field deal primarily with PTSD (e.g., Andrews, Brewin, Philpott, & Stewart, 2007; Solomon, 1993; Solomon & Mikulincer, 2006; Yehuda, McFarlane, & Shalev, 1998). No studies were found that focus on the impact of military service on young Israeli men in the years immediately following discharge, or of their later service as reservists or volunteers.

As noted by Danny Brom,[3] in a conversation we held in 2014:

> All the studies focus on PTSD. They found that between 15% and 28% suffer from PTSD, but the bigger question is: what does that mean relative to the others, since the myth is that you either have PTSD or nothing, which, of course, can't be right. I'm not familiar with publications that examine the sequentiality and talk about precisely what people who don't have PTSD actually are diagnosed as having, but that's exactly what's needed. In the Israel Center for the Treatment of Psychotrauma [ICTP] we give commando units questionnaires . . . and we see that 22% report symptoms that indicate PTSD, and about 25% that don't, but the rest, around 50%, are on that axis, and they are the ones to whom no one relates.

When I asked whether focusing only on PTSD serves as a kind of defence of avoidance from coming into contact with the consequences of the situation in which we live and that influences our daily lives, Danny agreed with me:

> That's a way for society to say, "There are those who aren't okay, but we *are* okay, we're immune". It's a central motif in the "robust nation".

Hadas Glazer writes[4] that the stories and voices of "ordinary" commando soldiers are never heard. Her partner, Yaron Edel, who had been a company commander in the Second Lebanon War, found a picture on the internet of the evacuation of wounded soldiers from the Saluki Creek battle, which was one of the harshest of the war, with many injured and twelve killed. She describes how Yaron, who had been almost obsessively preoccupied with reconstructing the events of that battle, said that the photo precisely matched his memory. He had carried the memory alone for years, unable to share or describe what he had experienced to anyone but fellow soldiers. Through this single photograph she was able for the first time to see and understand the war that was both present and absent in her life, but so impactful on them as a couple.

> Yaron posted the image to Facebook and within just twenty-four hours they had received hundreds of photos of the battle from soldiers, an awesome photographic archive that seemed to gather itself from some internal force of attraction, without any effort on our part.

Glazer believes that these simplistic narratives hold some threat over the Israeli existence that wants to believe that the IDF is the best army in the world, the most moral, one that would never go to war unless there was good reason. There is no legitimacy for the small stories of the IDF as a humane army, multi-layered, vulnerable, with many weak points. She believes that the stories are not being heard at the political level, nor at the level of social and personal conduct, and that we do not know how to approach and open this subjcct.

Glazer was one of the founding members of a new movement, "Splinters", which invites soldiers and their families to talk even if they are not post-traumatic, emphasizing the need to process the emotional experiences they have been through. A thousand participants came to the movement's first event, held in Jerusalem on Memorial Day.

A second play by Yinon bar Shira, *What's Your Problem?*, relates to the same issue. As Yinon explained,[5] he felt lucky he had completed three years of active service as a commando without being injured, physically or mentally. Only some months later did he start experiencing a recurring dream in which *a mistake had occurred, and he needed to enlist again, and there was war.* He believes that in our country, whether we want to admit it or not, all of us are shell-shocked in some way or another. We all grow up with this permanent reality of wars, and the soldiers who come back from them are the friends and relatives of us all.

Following the Second Lebanon War, the ICTP reported that soldiers, whether in compulsory service or serving as reservists, were highly exposed to trauma and loss, and their mental health needs had not been met, except in extreme circumstances.

The Ezrat Nashim Hospital, in conjunction with the Hebrew University School of Social Work, established an overseas support workshop that brings discharged soldiers together in a relaxed atmosphere, allowing them to verbalize their emotions and to re-enter civilian life from a stronger stance. Yaron Edel noted that

> Some people had extremely complex experiences, but they continue functioning, they go to work, to university, they are in a couple relationship, though something's missing there. Something's affecting our quality of life. And when I say "our" it's not just us the commandos, it's also our spouses or partners, our parents. The phenomenon, or the ripple of the phenomenon, is broad. People think it will harm them if they talk, that it's a weakness. It's important that people know that it's okay to talk and share these experiences. It's an important thing to do.[6]

Shahar Adna, a commando from the Second Lebanon War period, participating with his team in one of the workshops, said:

> In the workshop I talked about an event from the time of the last war, and a lot of my team chose to talk about that same event. By the end, we understood that blaming yourself or thinking that you did something incorrectly wasn't just your own feeling . . . the picture becomes clearer. I knew my team for years, and this is the first time I saw all of them cry. Not just one guy. Everything came out there.

The interviewer of a programme on Israel's Channel 20 posed a question right after Operation Protective Edge: "Isn't it better to just let things subside?" The workshop's director Sasson Richbi's answer is consistent with psychoanalytic knowledge on the impact of unprocessed trauma:

> The black box we put aside draws on our energy. Repression is not just good. At deeper than the superficial level, it uses up our strength, in the area of couple relationships, personal life, relationships with children.

Uri Carmi, who experienced the death of two friends in his unit, demonstrated the impact of trauma of which he been unaware:

> Eighteen months after the war more or less, we went in for reserve duty. And there we're still the same unit, and everything's okay, it's all great. And in some military action we had to handle disruptions.

> It used to be I wouldn't bat an eyelid over things like that, because unfortunately I'd been shot at in the past, had rocks thrown at me. This time I dropped down on the spot, as though "who's listening to what's happening here?" and I realized I'd lost my self-confidence as a soldier.

Zehava Solomon, Liat Lev-Shalem, and Rachel Dekel (2007) investigated the links between exposure to a traumatic event, subsequent development of stress, and world assumptions of 348 soldiers who had participated in the Yom Kippur War. Of these, 164 were former prisoners of war and 184 had not been captured. It was found that despite no obvious differences, soldiers who suffered from psychic stress reported more negative world assumptions than those who did not suffer from psychic stress.

Interrupted maturation-development continuity

The sequence of events occurring while serving as a commando from age eighteen until discharge three or more years later does not allow the young Israeli adult to develop at his own rate or according to his personal needs. At the height of the maturation process he may be in senior high school, military service, or civilian life. At age eighteen, he leaves his protective home environment, enlists, and is required to adopt a military identity, with its typical characteristics of heroism, achievement, dissociation from emotions, ability to withstand pain, and display of omnipotence and rigor (Lieblich, 1989; Sasson-Levy, 2006).

Benny, who had served as a commando and had been discharged more than a decade ago, came to me for psychotherapy because of difficulty in coping with life situations linked to continued maturation and development, such as taking on responsibility in his job or becoming a father. Coping with military service repeatedly surfaced in therapy:

> "My experience as a cadet was that it was like a children's game. A lot of people have no idea it's real. I was so down because I didn't like the pretence of the uniform, and I didn't understand that weapons kill. The first time I realized they killed, I was in shock. *I felt that that's not me, that there's a disparity between the me inside and the me I'd become in the army. I disconnected from myself*. I feel that way today too, and it's super-scary: it puts me in a state of anxiety."

When discharged soldiers return to live at home, the old dynamics according to which the relationships with parents were shaped are renewed, although the anxiety over sons' lives that drove those dynamics has disappeared once the sons are safely discharged. The young men therefore remain "stuck" with dependency on the mother and on the father, with whom no real relationship has ever been built that would allow identifying with him and adopting his identity as a masculine role model, and the additional emotional dynamics described so far. Under such conditions, the son is often filled with feelings of inexplicable anger and aggression, which he finds hard to understand in himself.

This is true for Caleb, a discharged soldier who, when serving, took part in campaigns that led to the death of terrorists. After discharge, Caleb returned to his parental home before setting off on his "great trek", and following that he came to me for therapy. He is intelligent, with high capabilities in multiple areas, but he felt confused, lost, filled with aggression and severe anxiety. His relationship with his mother was symbiotic: she spoilt him and did everything for him. From his few descriptions of his father, my impression was of a silent type, conveying weakness and distanced from a position of influence in the family. In the psychotherapy session, Caleb first described his military actions and the battles that led to the death of terrorists, and he then recalled a dream in which *Arabs have penetrated the house in which he is sleeping, and he is constantly searching for ways of saving himself without killing them*. Following that description, he spoke of feeling distress over not knowing what is happening to him, experiencing internal disconnects. He felt aggressive towards his friends without any obvious cause—if he played football with them and one of them annoyed him, he felt murderous towards him, and likewise in other situations—even with strangers. His distress kept growing.

I wondered if the drive to kill, which is usually buried beneath numerous wholesome defences, was exposed during his military service and continued to roam free in the depths of his psyche, tormenting him. Presumably, despite it being rationally clear to Caleb that through killing terrorists he saved a lot of innocent people, the very fact of killing has him facing emotional conflicts too weighty to bear; it was therefore necessary in therapy to bring Caleb into an encounter with them: "Perhaps these thoughts surface in you because you have already killed?" Caleb's face froze for several moments, and then, slowly, one tear after another began to fall. Tears rolled down my cheeks too, as I became aware of the emotional burden with which Caleb and all our other commando children must cope. After crying silently for a brief while, and with his eyes focused on mine, Caleb asked quietly, "So, then, does that mean I can longer not know what I actually do know?" Very quietly I answered him, "No, it seems not."

After this session, a change began within Caleb that allowed coming into direct contact with, and treating, places that previously had been obstructed, and this was accompanied accordingly by changes in his aggressive reactions.

The influence of emotional processes undergone by soldiers in active service can surface in civilian life years later. This is true for Dor, who adopted the commando identity fully and felt it was his true identity. He adapted well to his unit and its role, and he excelled, but on discharge found himself feeling empty. He then devoted three years to psychoanalytic therapy, during which he was able to complete previously unfinished developmental processes:

> "Before the army, I was weak, influenced by the environment. I didn't manage to bring myself to a state where I felt 'this is me'. I never found my voice. Even before the army, I never let myself rebel. I was always really close to my mother. The army is the cut, a trauma. Now I feel that the absence of freedom I agreed to in the army was unnatural, on the verge of dangerous. I felt like a baby playing in a theatre in the real world. I was really scared."

Dor set out on a fascinating journey of revelation and acknowledgment of his emotional layers, his authentic voice, the worlds that attracted him, discovering his abilities and strengths as well as his weaknesses, and coping with bringing these diverse facets into his personality to the point of integration into his "me". The symbiotic patterns typifying his childhood relationship, in which the experience of "the total fusion" and the "ultimate relationship" always require that one party negate her/himself in favour of the other, changed into patterns typical of a relationship between two people where each has a separate and unique identity. The change required him to invest work in the most important relationships in his life. On completing therapy, he said with a smile: "I came in feeling as a child who became a brave soldier, and I'm going out feeling almost a man."

These young adults clearly undergo powerful, if not extreme, physical and emotional experiences during their military service, and on discharge they must cope with complex emotional states. Like Caleb, along with the thrill of being discharged, they may experience suppressed, forceful urges of aggression and killing contrary to their values and about which, without battle action, they would have remained unconscious. In chapter seven, I reported Nadelson's (2005) findings that when commandos are discharged, they must cope not only with the knowledge that they are capable of killing, but that they actually experience pleasure from killing; they find difficulty in integrating these aspects into their personalities.

During military service they must cope with their own actions in war, with the death of mates, friends, and relatives; they must also often deal with ambivalence within Israeli society relative to their actions in the army, and often feel isolated because of the obligation of secrecy. In the army they must be disciplined: lack of obedience inherently carries harsh outcomes, from the danger of being killed, wounded, or taken captive to being punished according to military disciplinary guidelines, or being ostracized within their unit. Simultaneously with these tough requirements, Israeli soldiers function in a system of absolute dependence that dictates their daily agenda to the finest detail, thereby releasing them from the need to be independent. Once discharged, they must adopt a masculine civilian identity the characteristics of which are entirely different from those of the military.

When the young Israeli enlists, he is still dependent on his parents. The transition into the military framework is so sharp that multiple unconscious defence mechanisms are often aroused to deal with an emotional task that is beyond the psyche's natural ability to contain. This may in part manifest as the soldier feeling that his civilian personality is in constant conflict with his military personality. Should he have difficulty in containing this conflict, he may find himself in a state of psychic split: adopting everything required of him in the army while dissociating from his previous identity; repressing softer parts of his self, including emotions not suited to military life; and structuring a "false self" that adopts mannerisms of the commando male outwardly without connecting to his authentic internal world.

As Winnicott explained:

> If, in the fantasy of early growth, there is contained *death*, then at adolescence there is contained *murder*. Even when growth at the period of puberty goes ahead without major crises, one may need to deal with acute problems of management because growing up means taking the parent's place. *It really does.* In the unconscious fantasy, growing up is inherently an aggressive act. And the child is now no longer child-size. [Winnicott, 1971, p. 144; emphasis in original]

Winnicott's explanation sheds light on the difficulty experienced by every adolescent who has to cope with the meaning of murder enfolded into the process of normal growing up. From this, one can understand how difficult it is for the adolescent to cope when that period of growing up also includes experiencing himself as a real murderer. Not only is he no child, as Winnicott notes, he really can murder, and has.

Gidon, a discharged soldier, said:

> "I disgust myself. I wasn't like that before the army. I don't know how to *not* make others do things. A kind of manipulating them. Sometimes suddenly I'm sick of it all. Suddenly, for instance, I feel like I don't know my girlfriend Sara, the one I know, and she isn't herself. Suddenly I feel distanced from her, someone's there between us, a wall."

To my question, "What happens inside you in that instant when everything changes?" Gidon replied:

> "It's a second when I can't hold my walls up any more. I don't know if my arms get tired and everything comes down on me, and then everything's different, or it's something I go into . . . if it's falling down on me, I'm passive, it takes me over, a kind of anxiety, and changes my whole way of looking at things; fear can do it. I don't know what I want. Now, when I'm talking to you about Sara, *I can't see that 'I've got the soul' to do what has to be done,* it doesn't go into my brain . . . drives, maybe call it. When I don't give in to the drives I get anxiety attacks from it, as if I'm ignoring myself. At work I can watch porno movies for an hour and a half, and the boss thinks I'm one of his really good employees. What a poor thing he is, having the wool pulled over his eyes like that. I relate to him like my commander in the army. I fool him, I'm scornful of him."

Difficulty with emotional regulation and with adaptation are just two aspects of the difficulties of transition from military service to civilian life. The former is a whole world of adventures, full of challenging, exhilarating, powerful experiences; these are cut off suddenly on the day of discharge, the sudden switch catapulting the commando into civilian existence.

During his military service, the young Israeli commando often finds himself involved in complex missions that require courage and a sense of adventure, using expensive, complex equipment: tanks, ships, submarines, fighter jets, helicopters, highly advanced tools. Experiences may include diving, flying, parachuting, and more. His peers in the Western world would be unlikely to have encountered such things.

The experience of firing a gun is enormously powerful. The excitement comes first and foremost from the body (libido) with its pre-action alertness followed by accelerated heartbeat. The recoil effect first impacts the shoulder and then moves into the rest of the body. Some soldiers become addicted to these reactions and want to shoot at any opportunity. The weapon is experienced as an extension of the body. A soldier who has heard bullets whistling past his head will also testify that before the panic, the rationalization, there is excitement, especially with tracer bullets at night. Added to all the above is mutual responsibility for the lives of everyone in the unit.

During military service the young soldier is often allowed to use his judgement when it comes to firearms training sessions costing large amounts of money, but, more importantly, he uses his judgement when it comes to responsibility towards the lives of others. Ido and Ziv (see chapter seven) related to this succinctly in a conversation we held following Operation Protective Edge. Ido noted:

> "I don't understand how guys, after being in the army as commanders or officers, can go and work as waiters. It drives me nuts . . . If you'd done something not meaningful in the army, ok, I understand. But if you've served as a commando, and especially if you've commanded other soldiers, you've had people subordinate to you, suddenly to be a kind of "just you" that's not important to anyone . . ."

Often during military service there is a change in the way the soldier perceives himself on encountering responsibility, his functioning in a battle, and the complex range of experiences brought into play, all of which cause him to develop and attain unique capabilities. However, on discharge there is no continuity: he begins his life as though he had just completed senior high school.

I asked them: "What do you think about yourselves prior to recruitment and now, after these experiences?" Ido said that the change started with preparations before the war, but the fighting itself also changed a lot. Ziv added that the army enabled him to think in a more mature way on the big picture, not just about himself.

Ido detailed how in the army there's less room to shirk responsibility. Also, all the transitions in the army—from cadetship to advanced training, to commando units, to advanced courses, with people around you changing all the time—give you a lot of opportunity to change the less good things in yourself, because you're not taking up just one place in society.

Ziv said he felt that he had changed because he'd wanted to and allowed himself to. Military service gave him the option of maturing and looking at things differently. He concluded: "It depends on the person. A lot of people don't intend to let the army influence them, behave like kids, stay the same, and don't advance."

How can we expect an adolescent whose recruitment into the army created an intervention in his maturational process, whose life was directed by the army and who then suddenly finds himself a civilian, to continue consolidating his masculine identity in a natural way?

The lack of awareness in society of this complex emotional task conveys a mistaken message to the Israeli commando. He has difficulty in consolidating his identity, in finding his authentic self. The message he receives is that this is not a natural difficulty in the circumstances of Israeli existence but, rather, something that is problematic and damaged in him, leading to his feeling of loss.

Another aspect of the difficulties felt by the discharged combat soldier is tied to the structure of relationships created from birth between himself and his parents, and the effect on his personality.

Guilt and compensation as components in the structure of the parent–son relationship

As the interviews show, anxiety over a son's future recruitment accompanies the boy's life as he grows up, arousing in parents emotional patterns of ambivalence towards the birth of a son, helplessness relative to the parents' inability to change this reality, and feelings of guilt that shape parental patterns of compensation and overprotectiveness. These relationship patterns are deepened during the course of sons' military service, since they find themselves entirely dependent on the military framework and on support at home. This dynamic contradicts the natural developmental needs for independence and can create an experience of anxiety, inexplicable aggression, and confusion, as Gidon, who returned to live with his parents after discharge, explained:

> "At home, I'm just not capable of helping my mother. I simply can't. If I do that, I'm in a nightmare, or I'll go nuts . . .
>
> There's something really destructive in me, and if I give in to it, it'll make me poor, turn me into a drug addict . . .
>
> Maybe I simply want to do nothing, be forlorn, embitter my parents' lives until they die, always be my mother's child, and she'll always give in to me. I used to think *someone needs to get sick of me.* If only that would happen! Maybe my father will be able to do so eventually if my mother makes his life miserable because of me."

I interpreted that the feeling of destruction in him, connected to his wish that his mother and father would release him from dependency on them and allow him to build himself, has joined with the feeling of being able to destroy brought to light in the army, and together they are threatening to destroy him inside. And that's what he is fighting. Gidon responded:

> "The limit, because of my mother's attitude, I drew in my imagination, but I can't seem able to implement it. I've told you several times that I'm violent—that's exactly the issue. I feel that the more we go deeper inside, I'll find the fucking kingdom of the devil . . ."

Gidon's scream for his father to fulfil the developmental role that did not occur is clearly heard—the role that would draw a boundary to his childish behaviour and turn him into a "man". Faced with his inability to do so, Gidon imagines how he might bring the habits of dependency created by his parents to extremes—and especially bring his mother to her limit, so that, distressed, she will ask Gidon's father to fill that role and stop their son. In psychoanalytic terms, we can see the son's distress when the parents prevent him from successfully resolving the oedipal conflict. Gidon is typical of a large number of young men who come to my clinic following military service with similar emotional difficulties.

It is important to understand how complex these difficulties impacting everyday life are. Because patterns of ambivalent relationships, helplessness to save the son from the imminent danger of death, guilt, and compensation have often existed from before the son's birth, they *have become a part of the structure of the relationship between parents and son—in other words, a structural part of parenting, which creates secondary benefits for the sons and for the parents, who find it increasingly difficult to change this dynamic.* In this way, for example, the sons do not need to cope with the difficulties of independent life, and the parents do not need to cope with the "empty-nest" stage—a process that demonstrates their aging and approaching death.

The seepage of these processes into the relationship between the soldier and his commander enhances the secondary benefits—for example, in the form of easements in training that derive from parental intervention, or the relationship between the son at home on leave as someone "who deserves the best of everything", and more. The outcome is that this dynamic, instead of being weakened, becomes rooted in the relationship between parents and sons.

This dynamic, which becomes part of the sons' relationship structure and personality, is founded on one important component: parental anxiety over the death of sons during military service. But on discharge from the army, when it becomes clearly apparent that the son was not killed, *this central component in his emotional structure and the relationship between himself and his parents disappears*. The sons and parents together are "stuck" in the dynamic of mutual dependence, but in conditions different from those that created it. Parental anxiety and its accompanying benefits, which can no longer stake their claim on danger to the sons during military service, seek an alternative basis that will allow the continuation of the relationship and the emotional structure. For this reason, it is exchanged for dangerous forms of "the great trek", such as Peru's death road or bungee-jumping from clifftops. Of course, not all treks are like this. Some backpackers choose to spend most of their time lying about in guesthouses smoking grass; others go on a trip, come back, and continue their lives. But there is no doubt that for some the attraction of risk—which is the death drive—and excitement derive from the recent military past, through the exposure to violence and real risk of death.

This complex situation is followed by the confusing paradox that arises during combat service. Implementing difficult military operations and upholding the demanding requirements of an uncompromising system needs coping abilities and places weighty responsibility on the soldiers, all of which indicate some degree of maturity. All these traits have real value in personality-building. The outcome is no empty mask or veneer.

In Western societies in general, and in Israel in particular, the characteristics of masculinity parallel those of the commando (Sasson-Levy, 2006). However, since this often refers to a personality adopted without any integrative connection to earlier developmental stages, a self develops that is not authentic, concealing those layers of psyche that do not match the masculine commando identity. The "false self", according to Winnicott (1960), is an unconscious defence mechanism to conceal the true self and protect it. The soldier and his environment will experience it as true, but deep within the psyche a disparity exists between "true self" and "false self", which creates unconscious unrest and a sense of distress.

This does not imply, however, a dichotomy between a "true self" that is good and a "false self" that is bad. Winnicott identified several types of "false self", starting from the most pathological and extreme: the false self that "presents itself" as true while the true self remains latent; however, in close relationships the false self begins to fail, since it lacks some certain essential. Less extreme is the false self that protects the true self but simultaneously acknowledges the true self as a potential that allows a secret life behind behavioural symptoms of illness, which attempt to hint at the existence of a latent true self. A state of health is reached when the false self seeks conditions that allow the true self to realize its potential; the danger, if those conditions are not found, is that the personality will be forced to organize a new psychic defence against the true self's being taken advantage of, which may include suicide as a last resort to avoid betrayal of the true self. In contrast, the closest possibility to health is when the false self is built on identification with others; the false self is represented by the organization of a polite social stance and appropriate behaviours based on the individual's ability to forego the experience of omnipotence, since achievement is a place in society that is impossible to reach or hold by virtue of the true self alone (Winnicott, 1960).

The disparities between the maturation processes of the young Israeli male expose him to the danger of developing a false self in a range of pathological dynamics and manifestations.

The Israeli backpacker

Young Israelis set out on their "great trek" and often, at the declarative level, state "I'm going for an unlimited time", "Don't know how long I'll be gone", etc. This statement already shows the ambition for negative freedom, for disconnection from all commitments and responsibilities. However, the atmosphere during the trek often continues the military atmosphere, including precision planning and repeated checking of their ability to withstand the difficulties while taking risks with their lives that, unfortunately too often, end in catastrophe (Ben-Ari, 1998; Lieblich, 1989; Noy, 2007), such as the death of two backpackers in a kayaking accident in Peru's dangerous Apurimac River. They had gone kayaking despite being aware of the numerous warnings and appeals not to go by families whose loved ones had died in the same river.

The tendency to try adventurous sports activities and seek thrills out of a sense of "fulfilling a social role and expectation to go on a trek" was found by Mevorach (1997; see also Noy, 2007) to be among the traits of young backpackers.

Matching this statement, we find many parents supporting these treks, and even paying for them, out of guilt feelings "because the poor thing served in the army, so he deserves it". The trek's risks leaves the component of "anxiety over the son's life" intact, and the parental feelings of guilt once again absolve them of the need to adopt a conflictual stance with their sons and oppose the risky journey. Their helplessness thus also remains intact, but within a current context. The same dynamic is reconstructed at the political level: Israeli backpackers know in advance that the State of Israel, through its foreign ministry and international embassies, is willing and ready to come to their aid in problem situations without a thought to costs. Policymakers do not intervene in advance and try to negate the legitimacy of, and support for, life-endangering activities by Israeli youngsters.

In a study begun in 2002,[7] I interviewed 19 Israeli backpackers in their early twenties, who met on their treks through Australia and New Zealand. The question I asked them all was, "Who are you, Israeli backpacker?", adding nothing more.

All the respondents were discharged commandos. Unlike women backpackers, who go trekking with fairly clear plans set in place for their return, most of these young men manifested confusion and a sense of having lost their way. They went on their trek "to find themselves", expecting they would know what they wanted to study or do when they returned. The most important experience of the trek for them was "being on my own", which they explained as "doing things without anyone telling me what to do or worrying about me, not the army, not parents". All spoke of their close relationship with parents, especially with mothers. Bari said "I'm my mother's son." Proudly he described his independence. He said he had paid for the trip from his army savings and, without sensing the contradiction in his further statements, described how his mother checks his account and, if necessary, she makes up the difference. He explained that when he goes to study, his parents will pay, because he's *"not studying just for myself, I'm also studying for them"*.

Sagi's story is touching: he sat hunched over and helplessly said that he's already at the end of his trip. When he'd started it, he thought that by the end, he'd know "who I am". He described being in a tiny apartment in New York, on drugs, wandering the streets, not knowing where he was or where he was going. "I was out of it. Lucky no one at home knew. It was a frightening experience." He concluded: "Now I'm in a much better state. But I have no clue what's next? Where am I going to from here, and how?"

I could sense the confusion, anxiety, and emotional distress. There was general agreement that the young men who travelled in Australia and New Zealand were in a better psychological state than those who went to India. As one of them said: "In India there are so many guys who are totally wiped out. They said they walk around doing nothing, smoking drugs, having sex indiscriminately, just passing the days . . ." Another added: "India's a place without time and without limits . . . it's a frightening experience." While they were talking, I thought of the mothers fighting the dimension of time and eliminating boundaries, and I wondered whether a connection existed between the two aspects.

The aspect of danger in "the great trek" was demonstrated by Amnon, who had served successfully as a commander in an elite unit involved in several risky operations. Like many, he had gone on a "head-clearing" trip, starting out travelling through Australia on a motorbike, oblivious to any dangers. On one occasion, he fell and was trapped under the bike until rescued by chance the following day by other travellers. In another incident, he joined up with a bunch of ranchers who caught wild oxen by isolating the weaker ones in the herd. He described his role:

> "My job was to isolate the weak bull by riding around it on the motorbike. The guys managed to get their ropes around it, and when I thought it was tied down, I got off the bike to take a look . . . suddenly I found myself tossed in the air and then flat on the ground. Luckily for me the ranchers managed to get control of the animal. This time I realized I'd gone overboard with things, and I could see that in fact I was continuing to endanger my life. I stopped."

This story can also be understood from a metaphorical angle, when Amnon noted that he "joined up with a bunch of ranchers who caught wild oxen by isolating the weaker ones". This explains the somewhat conformist Israeliness in general, and Israeli backpackers in particular: "To be and to do like the others, so that no one should, God forbid, think I'm weak." Therefore, these tests of bravery come into play, events that add the dimension of a rite of induction to the trek. It is as though in the army, the soldier did not have a chance to fully display his masculinity, so these events allow for a continuation. The attitude is that, for example, "if the other guys did rafting here, in this dangerous part of the river, then of course I will too!" This thinking derives from a mix of social pressure and internal fear of being alone and being seen as a wimp.

Noy (2007), who researched groups of backpackers, found that many were seeking a continuation of long-term physical exhaustion and tended to spend their time in enclaves of Israeli backpackers, looking for the lightest type of entertainment, seeking out "spiritual" experiences or using drugs, travelling for anything from several weeks to several years.

It may be that "the great trek" allows flight from encountering harsh memories, as Aaron described. He had fought in the Second Lebanon War and lost three of his soldiers in a fierce battle. He said that some of his team-mates went overseas and never returned to Israel, to avoid meeting the people or the unpleasant memories or making a decision about their futures. These are soldiers "stuck" in the past. Later, some of the unit members didn't show up for reserve duty as a way of avoiding the conflict with these memories, and they chose to cut contact.

Two contradictions surface from the interviews. First, it is puzzling why young men who have just been discharged safely from dangerous military service are willing to risk their lives again; second, it is no less puzzling that society expects this of them. Noy points to an additional contradiction. While the travellers claim they want to "rest", "find distance", "get some peace" from the pressuring and violent Israeli existence, their actions indicate that they make major efforts to placing a checkmark against yet another station along the path of Israeli life. They also endeavour to spend time with other Israelis in enclaves filled with the presence of Hebrew, shown in shop signs and restaurants.[8]

Seeking an explanation in the unconscious layers reveals a concealed emotional dynamic. It seems that these symptoms have become so deeply rooted because they serve simultaneously several unconscious, parallel, and contrasting emotional needs. Consciousness of its nature will serve as the first step towards developing the ability to join civilian life.

Two components of emotional stress among discharged soldiers—the need to distance from unprocessed traumatic memories, and the need to complete the process of consolidating an independent masculine identity, while completing the processes of separation from the mother and creating a renewed masculine identity with the father—lead to trekking. The withdrawal into trekking, mysticism, and blunting or numbing of senses allows "flight" from encountering the emotional burden that tortures, depresses, and arouses anxiety, created both as they grew up in the shadow of parenting patterns that did not support their masculine Israeli development and through the highly charged emotional situations in which combat soldiers find themselves, as described above. The source of this emotional charge is not apparent to the discharged soldiers, being for the most part unconscious.

Taking risks on their treks reinforces the masculine commando false self, at the basis of which is the childish protected personality, a false self that cannot continue to exist without continued military behaviours.

Distancing from the home, conducted at a superficial level in the service of the processes of separation–individuation, reveals itself beneath that level as an inverse rationale, since it actually continues the element of danger that upholds patterns typical of the parents' relationship for the duration of the sons' life: patterns of parental anxiety over their lives, helplessness in the face of their actions, and guilt feelings that overwhelm on the basis of "the child deserves a bit of freedom and to be supported and compensated". In this way, the act meant to complete masculine development creates a perpetuation of the dynamic of lack of separateness from the parents and non-completion of the developmental tasks, with the parents' full cooperation. In other words, the continued threat to the sons' lives allows that same unconscious dynamic between the sons and their parents that typified their growing up and shaped their personality and relationship with their parents to continue existing in a pattern of dependence, along with continued parental pampering. This means perpetuation of a disorder that occurred in the sons' separation–individuation processes. It preserves the only possible structure that exists: of dependence and sometimes even symbiosis. Without any other developmental process, sons will find difficulty in shaping their mature masculine "true self".

Undoubtedly, for some with sufficient ego forces, the trek represents a period in which an almost vital mediating stage occurs towards finding balance, recharging with new energy, and release. These young adults find the courage to decide, take action, and cope with freedom—no simple matter, after years of being in frameworks. The trip allows them this opportunity.

However, I view the phenomenon of trekking in its current format as a regressive phenomenon, which inhibits growth and development.

As noted, to date no in-depth study exists that observes both the conscious and unconscious layers, and I trust that this chapter will constitute the basis for further psychoanalytic research on this subject.

Notes

1. In regular compulsory service, after three years; for officers, after five to nine years.
2. https://www.youtube.com/watch?v=KSqJuQ4wcsA

3. Founder and director of the ICTP, in Jerusalem.

4. On the website Ellipsis.

5. On the official Hebrew website of the Kfar Saba Municipality (www.kfar-saba.muni.il/?CategoryID=255&ArticleID=5072), where the performance was presented.

6. From an article by Yasour Beit-Or, 19 April 2010, on the Hebrew website, Ynetnews.

7. This was a preliminary study of the processes undergone by the young Israeli male from the time he receives his first draft order, through combat service, to several years after discharge. The study was never completed, due to war.

8. From a 2009 article on Noy's Hebrew Facebook page, "The Wandering Israel" (www.bac.org.il/myvhdym/project/hatrmylaym/article/hayshraly-hanvdd).

CHAPTER NINE

The "peacetime self" and the "wartime self"

Clearly the interpretive description of the unconscious stages of Israeli masculinity presented so far is not the only one. Future studies focusing on other populations—various minorities sectors;[1] the ultra-Orthodox sector, which is exempt from conscription, although a few of them do enlist; military careerists; bereaved families with teenage sons; immigrant families, in which the parent generation was too old to serve but their sons do; and so forth—will no doubt depict more hues and shades of what it is to reach masculinity in Israel.

Nor does this study represent the narrative of *all* parents to sons in Israel, or the maturation stages of *all* Israeli combat soldiers. However, the narratives are shared by a meaningful proportion of Israeli society and hence influence the Israeli experience. An expanded public discourse is therefore needed on this topic if we are to gain a more complete picture that identifies the full dialectic impact of events that fill the Israeli reality, and the unconscious emotional processes.

The narratives and insights discussed may have created the mistaken impression that these individuals are flooded with psychological problems and are part of a sick society. But, as we know, an ideal world does not exist, not even in fables. A closer look at any society will reveal complex emotional dynamics, each with its own price and characteristics, requiring the appropriate ability to cope.

Uncovering emotional layers concealed because of trauma, while raising consciousness of uniquely Israeli patterns, may actually be a source of strength that creates the potential for personal, familial, and national space. Winnicott (1971) defined "potential space" as an area of the psyche that allows containment of the conflict, thought, and internal observation needed for growth and development. It exists between phantasy and reality and allows us the sense of healthy and recuperative selfness. The ability to contemplate and acknowledge what had previously not been possible releases some of the grip of these powerful unconscious forces in us and thereby lends us greater freedom of choice. The existence of potential space is vital to enabling adoption of parenting and couple-relationship patterns, as well as parents' and sons' personality structures that are able to contain the parts found in conflict, while conducting an internal discourse and integrative connection to internal and external realities. Moreover, a potential space of this kind may become a beneficial chain of influence from the individual to the general, and, finally, to the entire system.

Consciousness of the unconscious dynamic alone is not enough, however, to release an individual from its grasp. Means to enable continuity of the development process are discussed in chapter ten.

The peacetime self and the wartime self

In a 1919 article, Freud related to diverse personal expressions that manifest in times of peace compared with times of war:

> The conflict is between the soldier's old peaceful ego and his new warlike one, and it becomes acute as soon as the peace-ego realizes what danger it runs of losing its life owing to the rashness of its newly formed, parasitic double. [Freud, 1919, p. 208]

Freud related to everyone who experienced war, civilian or soldier, but especially to soldiers who undergo the jolting experience of war.

The soldier who has killed

The soldier's privilege to kill is unlike any other human experience, and he is ultimately changed, linked to the death he brought about. Years later, soldiers become agitated when remembering battle victories and the deaths involved. The primal terror on encountering the enemy, which changes with victory that follows the battle against death, is accompanied by an emotion never felt before and creates a moment frozen in time, differentiated from all other memories: a point of perspective on life (Nadelson, 2005). The experiences of soldiers during war cannot be divided into experiences of victory or experiences of defeat. It may be erroneously thought that the experience of victory in battle leaves no traumatic footprint in the soldier's psyche. But soldiers find themselves in a range of situations during war, creating a broad spectrum of emotional reactions. Thus, even if soldiers have experienced victory, for example, many moments exist in the overall experience of war which cannot connect with the attacking enemy, as noted in earlier chapters.

Nadelson (2005, p. 8) explained that when people experience an attack directed at them but are unable to protect themselves, they experience a state of emotional flooding that causes them to function automatically; the absence of a natural human reaction is oppositional to self-preservation. In contrast, when the soldier does have the option of effective action, he experiences extreme thrill. The experience of pleasure is the payback that is perhaps "hardwired" in our psyche through social and biological development, and this experience remains etched in soldiers' psyches even after their discharge.

The victory achieved, from the starting point of a life-endangering situation, remains etched in memory, bound in the feelings of fear and shock at seeing wounded or dead comrades. The battle over life and death will be remembered in future with feelings of satisfaction and joy, mixed with those of terror, distress at the loss of mates, and other memories of war, none of which can be truly forgotten (Nadelson, 2005, p. 79). The incidents presented in chapter seven testify to this phenomenon.

Helplessness is one of the conditions of trauma. The psyche reconstructs traumatic events in order to overcome them (Freud, 1920). Without sufficient emotional processing of these powerful experiences, the discharged soldier will, in order to blunt them, have to employ defence mechanisms such as repression or dissociation. The psyche is pulled in opposing directions: on the one hand, between memories of the extreme thrill of victory and avoidance of memories of terror, pain, and bereavement; on the other, drawn into memories of trauma in order to overcome them. This oppositional tugging can cause states of distress.

Attitudes to the law

The wartime psyche is also different from that of peacetime in its attitude to the law. In times of peace, the law is a pillar of civilization, and honouring it allows societies to reject revenge under all circumstances. But wartime enforces a different outlook on the cultured individual. Gratification and justice come through the gun and become absolute actions through automatic reflex. Thinking too much can cost the soldier his life. Soldiers are reflexively willing to give their lives to save their fellow soldiers. Their fury at the death of comrades and drive for revenge is unavoidable, and many cannot resist it: the pull for revenge overrides all other needs. It takes absolute control and creates a strong appetite for death. Nadelson (2005) described how soldiers who had fought in Vietnam afterwards felt they had been in a kind of hallucinatory state.

Many soldiers have experienced the death of fellow soldiers and friends in various situations: a soldier who died alongside the survivor; who died in a battle in which the survivor had not fought; who died saving the survivor's life; who died as a result of disregarding safety instructions, or conversely, who died because the survivor disregarded safety instruction; and many other scenarios. Obviously every soldier will therefore carry complex emotional baggage that will impact them during their lifetime.

The psychoanalysts Donald Winnicott and Wilfred Bion both experienced World War I, and the effects of this on them are reflected in their writings. Winnicott was a medical student in London when the war broke out; later he served as a surgeon on a destroyer. Many of his friends and acquaintances died because of the war. The influence of their deaths and his connection with them was his feeling of being part of a much larger body, its totality and form concealing far more than is revealed, like some kind of gigantic crystal. His second wife, Clare, testified that all his life, Winnicott was influenced by this feeling, and he always felt a sense of responsibility to live not just for himself but for those who had died (C. Winnicott, 1990). According to Christopher Reeves (2004), Winnicott's loss of friends during the war accompanied him throughout his life as unconscious trauma, and its footprint can be traced in his description of the emotional state of "fear of breakdown" (Winnicott, 1963).

Ogden (2014) states that Winnicott's "Fear of Breakdown" is a vague, incomplete paper. Winnicott wrote that in infancy, a mother–infant breakdown occurs that obliges the infant to digest emotional events that its psyche cannot organize. Experiences that did not undergo emotional processing continue to have a psychotic dissembled nature, and so the infant must put up a defence against it by creating an internal life reality that substitutes for the external reality containing the experience of the breakdown in the relationship with the mother. From that time on, the individual lives with unconscious anxiety over a breakdown that has actually already occurred but not been experienced.

Wilfred Bion, still a teenager, fought as a tank commander, was promoted to a higher rank, and even won a medal of valour. When his tank took a direct hit, he continued fighting in the open field, giving instructions to the other soldiers. Bion experienced himself as a soldier with no ability, and a tank commander with no chances. All his memories of the battle were horrific: he described a situation in which people had no idea where they were going, illogical orders were given that he termed "instructions to execute", and people were killed for no reason (Bion, 1997). For Bion, trauma was a form of residual memory of the tangible horrors of death and destruction in the battlefield. It seems he was attacked by these memories later in the classic form described by Freud as "revenants", which disabled his sense of purpose and his vitality and left him for the longest time unsure of his career and doubtful about his abilities in any sphere—in an authentic anxious-depressive state (Reeves, 2004). Bion's daughter Parthenope also raised the question of how, and to what extent, her father's personality as an analyst was shaped by his war experiences: she pointed to his interest in the simultaneous states of primitive regressed states together with protomental states (P. Bion Talamo, quoted in Jacobus, 2005).

These two examples illustrate the influence of war experiences continuing to be active in an individual's life, intertwined in life events, and difficult to identify.

There are, of course, abundant examples in Israel expressing the feelings manifest later in life by soldiers who experienced war. In his song "July August Heat", popular Israeli singer Shlomo Artzi describes a squadron passing through a wadi in the midday heat, "wounded, trembling". He describes the contradiction between beautiful youthfulness and military procedures and then returns to recording the scenes: "Floating on stretchers/two without names/Lately these images from there come back to me/In my faded current memories/a heavy curtain of wars and hallucinations." He ends by clarifying the difficulty of return to life's routine: "I'm going to dance with soldiers dead in their hearts."

In another song, "Unquiet Night", Artzi gives expression to feelings of guilt over being alive. These are very harsh feelings that recall to some extent those of Holocaust survivors. He describes how the wife of a friend who fell tempts him to sleep with her, and he dreams about the friend: "I wake because I dreamt how they/they're shooting at you, they hit you and you're crying." The singer tries to console himself with the thought: "Perhaps you've found the rest/among soldiers you're allowed", followed by: "I take solace and sleep with her/as though filling in for you."

Israeli reality overflows with images of this nature, starting with the bodies of dead Egyptian soldiers in the sands of Sinai, all the way through to soldiers crawling on all fours through the dirt on the Philadelphi Corridor on the Israel–Gaza border, seeking "their friends".

Euphoric joy can be a mark of mourning. Exposure to shedding blood can lead to nihilism, apathy, mania, as well as to feelings of euphoria and omnipotence that "nothing can damage me now that I've encountered death". Conversely, it can cause withdrawal, to the point of clinical depression, or severe aggression, as Freud (1915c) explained, in the form of anger towards the self that manifests as aggression directed outwardly, a wish for self-penalization that can develop into violence towards other people and even animals.

Discontinuity: the unspoken heritage of wars

With normal life suddenly interrupted by military service, and later continued without the link to its starting point, discontinuity becomes the unspoken heritage of war, constituting a central emotional component that binds the totality of understandings detailed in this book.

This inherent damage is evident in Richard Hughes's 1961 story, *The Fox in the Attic*, with its conclusions about experiences of the generation raised in World War I—a process that seems, surprisingly, wholly relevant to Israeli society. The narrative's protagonist, Augustine, growing up during World War I, simply accepted a world of war as normal. Children of his generation could barely remember what had previously existed and couldn't imagine that one day the war would cease. Children knew that, in all likelihood, they would not live much beyond nineteen, and they accepted that as the natural order of things—like the biblical three score years and ten. In church they heard the names of the fallen and accepted this as their reality. Sometimes it was a family member, and this would for a moment bring them closer to the thought that killing is radical, not like the gradual fading away of the elderly (Hughes, 1961). Then, when Augustine was eighteen, the war ended. His shock was tremendous: no one had warned him about needing to live a full life, with sixty years at his disposal, instead of the mere six months he had been certain was all the time available to him. Peace was an unknown and terrifying state he could not even imagine. The entire reality in which he had grown up and matured had melted away.

The parallel with Israel's reality is chilling: *the protective parenting patterns, which interfere and compensate, are a cover-up for transmission of parental anxiety to and onto their sons*. What appears to be "protection" of sons is actually "usage" of the son in order to be rid of feelings of anxiety while transmitting the message of the likelihood that he would die in war. These social messages throughout the sons' lives, from kindergarten to final year of senior high, powerfully keep the deaths of Israel's war fallen alive for the young Israeli, and perhaps also for those who take heritage trips to Holocaust concentration camps, which experientially allow living the Holocaust's events. Taken together, all these factors create the unconscious knowledge in sons, and perhaps also in parents, that sons will die at eighteen. In fact, parents have said this openly when describing and trying to create for their sons a world that is "all good", because "who knows what might happen later". Several parents described sons who expressed fears about the army or showed symptoms such as clinginess to parents (chapters two and three). The parents linked this to anxiety in their sons when the latter grow up. It would seem that the sons internalize this message.

The discharged sons later find themselves facing decades of life for which they are unprepared. Moreover, their relationships with their parents are rife with anxiety, guilt, and dependency, and these do not support necessary change. This dynamic occurred without knowledge of the sons' future military service—hence, all the processes described above were also activated in the sons. Clearly, it is therefore easy to feel lost after discharge from the army. However, most Israeli men do "find themselves" and function as masculine Israelis: we find successful young men at the cutting edge of science, technology, academia, and creative productivity, and filling diverse roles in family and society. It is important to establish whether success in these various areas of life correlates with emotional health and what made it possible for them to reach these desirable positions in Israeli reality, in order to assist those who are not able to complete the emotional developmental task of consolidating a separate masculine identity.

Note

1. Minorities are integrated into meaningful, though voluntary, service in the IDF. A large percentage of serving Druze reach very high command ranks. Most of the Assyrian population serves in the IDF, and several hundred Bedouin and Arabs enlist every year.

PART III

STEPS TOWARDS AMELIORATION

CHAPTER TEN

Psychoanalytic interventions

We have seen how raising sons with the knowledge of their future recruitment and military service itself have numerous consequences on shaping the mind and relationships of the individual, the couple, and the family. The psychoanalytic theory behind this related to individuals and families has also been outlined. Should, however, psychoanalysts hold an interventionist role in the national and international arenas at the level of theory, and perhaps even practice?

Taking a stance for the practical application of psychoanalysis is not new. In 1932, Alfred Einstein, fearing that the fate of nations was in the hands of entirely irresponsible political legislators, invited Freud on behalf of the League of Nations[1] to discuss whether there is a way of delivering mankind from the menace of war. In his response, Freud noted the central role of life and death drives in managing the psyche and therefore in managing personal and international life. He concluded that if the willingness for war is the outcome of the drive for destruction, then using Eros—destruction's opposing force—would help combat it; therefore, any factor contributing to the establishment of emotional links among humans should be actively involved against war (Freud, 1933, p. 211). He further added that through emotional affinity and other emotional sharing, which form the basis of human society, it is possible to counter the tendency to aggression. He noted that it would not be utopian to hope that anxiety itself over the outcomes of war, and all factors that promote the development of culture, should contain what it takes to work against war. Nonetheless, he qualified his statements by noting that human aggression could be restrained only through the existence of a central authority with "the last word" on any international dispute.

The very fact that Freud attempted to apply his theoretical understandings to political and international affairs must, in my view, challenge psychoanalytic therapists to continue his approach. It is incumbent on psychoanalysts in general, and those specializing in couple and family psychoanalysis in particular,[2] to contribute their expertise to a public understanding of the impact of unconscious processes on conduct in society.

I first summarize the analytic understandings presented so far and then propose suggestions for psychoanalytic intervention.

Emotional flooding. The source of the intrapsychic and interpersonal emotional dynamics' "entanglement" in mothers, fathers, and sons is emotional flooding, with loss anxiety and aggression, as well as unconscious guilt feelings. These draw simultaneously from two layers: the Israeli reality of compulsory military service, and intergenerational trauma mingled with current trauma. Their conjunction strengthens them until parents find it impossible to contain them, which causes the activation of multiple defence mechanisms. This dynamic spreads areas of influence via the interaction of parents with the education system and, later, with the military system. Moreover, through parents' involvement in both systems, these operate under the same unconscious conditions, and so the same dynamics seep into both.

Basic coping mechanisms. The basic mechanisms used to cope with this emotional background are projective identification and introjective identification—that is, processes of *splitting, projection, internalization,* and *identification.* This is what is called "a couple state of mind": an emotional dynamic produced through unconscious cooperation, where in mutual dynamics each psyche splits the two parts of the conflict it cannot contain and projects half onto his or her partner, who internalizes that part and identifies with it. In this way, each receives an "identity" based on the half of the conflict she or he "owns". The couple relationship turns into one between two parts of the conflict—in short, a conflictual relationship. Actually, each partner in the couple relationship functions as though half of a whole. This creates unidimensional behaviour patterns in the couple that, without regulation, become powerful.

In contrast, when the mind contains the conflict, one side of it regulates the other, and together they give the psyche contact with the complexity of the conflictual issue. The internal discourse between the components creates movement, change, and development. In such a state, each person comprising the couple is a whole person, and the discourse between the two, with each coping with the emotional conflict, allows mutual support, finding conscious solutions together and, especially, relations of intimacy, movement, and development.

This outcome is a response to the emotional flooding, allowing personality integration and a complex discourse at the personal and family levels relative to schooling and the military. If this principle is clear, it can be translated into action at the personal, familial, institutional, and national levels. Perhaps this is where the opening lies for a different mode of observation of international relations.

I now offer some initial thoughts on suggestions for intervention in the context of the Israeli situation.

Parents

Support groups for parents of sons and/or psychoanalytic couple therapy

Raising awareness and understanding

It is important to raise awareness, particularly among parents, of the emotional processes that impact Israeli parenting patterns relative to sons, and their effect on couple relationships and on the sons themselves. Simultaneously, it is also worth examining how this dynamic impacts the raising of daughters. Awareness is vital for better balance and stability in parental function. Conscious parents may function less as "marionettes" that operate under powerful unconscious forces and thus gain better control over their lives. Raising awareness must come about through the media, through education (seminars, courses to train educators), through therapeutic groups, and at the level of decision makers.

Psychological working through

Awareness of emotional processes on their own is not sufficient to create change in parenting, and may even confuse and cause harm. What is needed is "emotional work" by each parent and as a couple on containment options and reactive mechanisms. Through therapy as a couple—particularly the psychoanalytic couples approach, which relates simultaneously to each parent's unconscious dynamic and the way they structure the unconscious of the couple dynamic—both parents will be able to process the conflict that caused confusion over parenting in the other's presence, and together the couple will be able to create a balanced relationship with the son and offer the range of required parenting functions. Because these powerful emotions shared by so many parents encompass anxiety over their sons' lives, ambivalence towards them, helplessness, and guilt feelings, which in the current situation are transmitted to and onto the sons, a forum of support groups for parents of sons would be needed, facilitated by professionals trained for this very purpose and/or for working in psychoanalytic couples therapy in order to process the *emotional continuity and division of roles into which parents of sons feel thrust*, as shown in the current study.

Processing new parental patterns

In addition to emotional processing, support groups should assist parents in shaping patterns of resilience-focused/oriented parenting (Lewow, 2004) that will allow the space needed for the son's development in the relationship between himself and his parents. Parents will be able to gain integrative communication skills when each contains the totality of conflictual emotions. In this way, the relationship can become a place of discourse, support, learning, and partnership—one that supports growth and development, not only of each person involved, but also of the couple and the whole family. Parents will be able to raise a son while protecting his life and simultaneously encouraging the separation–individuation processes and, at the same time, supporting consolidation of his Israeli identity, including its commando components. The son, for his part, will not receive dual contradictory messages or the message that being a man threatens his mother or his father, his parents as a couple, or his own life. Parents who avoid conflictual stances and are in a mutual process of change and development may constitute a model for a healthier relationship for their son, who can thus learn how to conduct a relationship that includes negotiation, discussion, agreement, disagreement, and support—one in which one can belong and be connected, with a unique identity.

Supporting the son's path to masculine development

The maturation of many sons is accompanied by split rather than balanced parenting: a supportive but silent father and a dominant, resistant mother. A parent who can contain anxiety over a son's life can assist his encounter with the present reality, without any surplus or imagined emotional baggage. Since a boy's development includes military service at eighteen, parents who can support their son's masculine consolidation process can also, together with him, encounter the fear of military-sourced injury or death from a realistic place, along with the calming knowledge that the vast majority of recruits do not die, but develop unique capabilities and become men. An example of a complex yet balanced message created in this way is conversation about the military: how the son can contribute to the country, and how the military track will serve him later in civilian life. This allows the son to cope with fear, receive palliative messages that the army is one stage in his development, and acknowledge the values of giving to others while simultaneously realizing personal gain.

Acknowledging the son's military service as a contribution to parents, family, and society

When anxiety over the son's life is contained by parents and not transferred onto the son, the moment of enlistment becomes not a feeling of loss of life but, rather, the "empty nest" stage of natural development.

Acknowledging that the chance of their son being killed during military service is very low requires parents to contain anxiety, including intergenerational anxiety, and reduce the intensity of guilt feelings also transmitted intergenerationally. Such an integrative emotional state allows parents to convey to their son, in addition to blessings for his safety and good health in this new stage of his life, the understanding that he is about to receive effective tools for guarding his own life, and also to convey acknowledgment of his masculinity, capabilities, and the importance of giving to family and society through the act of enlistment.

This kind of message can be given only by parents who relate to their son as a man capable of protecting others: he thus receives the acknowledgment of his masculinity and maturity that he so greatly needs at this age.

Schools

Parental hostility towards schools versus partnership in the educational journey

Currently the *basically hostile attitude* among parents—*particularly mothers—to school* arises from emotions that view school as yet another framework anticipating the son's removal from them and bringing his possible death through military service yet closer. This situation causes frequent, harmful parental intervention in schools' actions and prevents constructive parental criticism regarding studies or the educational staff. Were schools aware of this attitude, they could help parents to contain these complex emotions, begin altering their approach to the school, and create new patterns of communication between parents and school. Parents who can contain their feelings of anxiety, guilt, and aggression will be able to identify the school as a place that provides their son with opportunities for development, freeing the educational staff to deal with educational activities.

Orientation towards constructive achievement

As education must prepare young Israelis for their unique life tasks, including military recruitment and discharge followed by continued civilian life, it is important for schools to do a *thorough check of their educational stances,* between on the one hand emphasizing "fun" and "enjoyment" and lowered demands for achievement and, on the other, turning the school into a "factory for high grades". For the first type of school, it is important to examine whether these leniencies derive from a dynamic of split between loss anxiety, guilt, and, possibly aggression, which are unconsciously expressed within the school and should be appropriately addressed. As for the second type of school, it is important to ensure that emphasizing achievement is not a form of avoidance of encountering the emotional world of the student who must enlist on completing his studies. Integration of open approaches to the many emotions accompanying the young Israeli's maturation with his preparation for military life should be the guiding light of every Israeli school.

Processes of separateness and uniqueness

Empowered *independence* is a vital component in the maturation process, expressing separateness and individualism. Therefore, fostering it should be included in the school programme by gradually placing increasing responsibility on students and simultaneously encouraging their independence.

Acknowledging the pre-recruitment stage

The education system should acknowledge that its senior-high-school students are involved in army recruitment processes during their final year of studies, and this will affect their preparation for matriculation examinations, which should therefore be moved to the close of Year 11. This would allow students to devote their final year of school to academic, emotional, social, and value-based content, creating a bridge between school, military service, and their futures following military discharge. This function is increasingly adopted by pre-military colleges, where senior-high-school graduates spend the year before recruitment studying leadership, democracy, contribution to the community, conceptual and ethical identity consolidation, Zionism, Judaism, philosophy, social activism, and many other areas.

Commemorative and mourning days

Holocaust Day and Memorial Days for Israel's fallen transmit parents' and teachers' intergenerational trauma and uncontained anxiety. Psychoanalysts should examine how these events are observed in educational institutions.

The messages transmitted to children, from kindergarten to senior high school, should be examined for continued emotional processing, symbolization, and mentalization—that is, for emotional processing of the powerful raw content, while emphasizing separation of past from present. Thus, it is necessary to avoid recreating trauma that can unconsciously take control of the psyche, preventing it from discerning the unique conditions of a current threat and, instead, mistakenly conflating it with past threats of extinction. Moreover, rituals of death and melancholy should be avoided, to prevent nurturing the view that only the dead are heroic. The concentration of sorrowful stories and accompanying testimonies of death may lead boys to the unrealistic assumption that it is their destiny too. It may additionally lead to nihilism, fear of the military, and depression or may encourage political extremes of nationalism or the far left, neither of which shapes mature opinion: they only indicate the adolescent's unresolved emotional conflict. Manipulative and demagogic use for short-term political purposes of ideological and populist elements of Israel's war fallen and Holocaust victims should be avoided.

The army

Gradual transition from military to civilian life

Observing the current disparity between the military and civilian worlds shows the need for the IDF or another government body to create a system that enables discharged soldiers to transition gradually from one world to the other.

While they are in the army, soldiers are told where to sleep, where to eat, what to do throughout the day. Advancement in the army brings more freedom, space, and responsibility, yet their basic needs—food, lodging, activities, belonging, and security—are still provided. Zak described how, on discharge, he hadn't a clue where to go or what to do, which credit card to get, what career to follow, etc.: "They just tell you to go figure things out yourself."

In light of such sharp transitions after discharge, a programme is needed covering the general issues that comprise adult civilian life: educational and professional options, academia, sport, culture, family life, democracy, and filling in income tax returns, national insurance, etc. The programme could be offered after discharge in a mentorship or group format, meeting regularly each week, to provide backup in practical areas as well as emotional processing of the transition.

The programme operated by the ICTP (see chapter eight) could be viewed as a starting point for structuring additional programmes. The centre sends groups of commandos overseas for a period of emotional processing and preparation for the future; participants indicate that the programme allows them to re-enter civilian life far more emotionally ready.

These are initial ideas intended to arouse further thought and implementation.

Society at large

Current threat versus past threat of annihilation

It is important to be aware that because states of threat relative to the country from hostile factors magnetize intergenerational trauma to current anxiety, undigested expressions of threat from the past become manifest. In this way, media and politicians are influenced by unconscious forces that maximize anxiety and distress and mask the ability to think and react proportionately. The threats belong in the present, but the strong emotional reaction to them is, partly, a reaction to trauma from the past. Freud (1914) stated that the patient experiences trauma as a real event in the present, and it is for analysts to do the work that manifests to a great extent in returning things to their past origins. During Operation Protective Edge, for example, news clips were shown repeatedly of a missile, fired towards the centre of Israel, bursting in mid-air: very few missiles took that path, but the impression was that dozens of them had. Similarly, repeated clips of sirens being activated in various locations in Israel made it seem as though all of Israel heard sirens several times each day.

Summary

The layered insights revealed in this study lead us to acknowledging the importance of emotional integration capable of containing conflictual worlds and powerful emotions; similarly, that unprocessed trauma from earlier generations, experienced powerfully in the current generation, can mistakenly be attributed to events in the present. It also highlights the need for a public psychoanalytic stance on these.

The separation between content that individuals carry in their psyches, in terms of "my content" versus "not-my content", the latter being the unconscious transmission of intergenerational trauma, makes it easier to understand—and thereby contain—the emotional picture. An integrative emotional position is beneficially impactful at several levels:

» *At the personal level,* it promotes good mental health while allowing development and creativity—the vital conditions for success and prosperity.

» *At the cognitive level,* it prevents wasting energy on maintaining defence mechanisms, leaving the greater portion of internal resources for learning and development, thereby allowing individuals, couples, and families to realize their abilities.

» *At the social level,* it fosters a frank encounter with reality, correctly evaluating the level of threat, and adapting the reaction proportionately. This, in turn, allows reaching achievements in the most precise way possible.

Containing powerful emotions serves to block emotional flooding by society and its institutions. It allows society to avoid being blindly jolted by the burden of its past and, instead, be more creative, directed to a higher quality of life and achievement. A society that focuses on the present while remembering the past and directing itself towards the future is one in which the individual can accept its conditions, and the need for belonging and vitality, without loss of identity. It is a society that can accept the other and its different parts and is therefore a healthy society—one that can identify threats of war and protect itself on the one hand, while identifying opportunities for peace and taking advantage of them on the other.

Notes

1. The League of Nations became the basis for the current United Nations.
2. In 2006 the International Association of Couple and Family Psychoanalysis was established. A year later, an international training programme in couple psychoanalysis was founded under the auspices of David Scharff, in which psychoanalysts and psychotherapists from the USA, London, and Israel participate; the Israeli psychoanalytic training programme was founded and led by the author.

APPENDIX

Research method

In this Appendix, I describe how and why the couples were chosen for the study, how the interviews were conducted, and the methods applied for analysing and interpreting the data. As the interviews have drawn a new picture of Israeli parenting, this should help the reader to follow the path along which these understandings arose from the text.

The research question

The basic premise behind the research was that, from the time a couple in Israel learns that their unborn child will be a son, conscious or unconscious anxiety surfaces throughout the child's life from the knowledge that, at age eighteen, he will be drafted into military service.

Wishing to examine this premise, a preliminary study was conducted, as outlined in chapter one. On the basis of the findings from this, it was possible to rely on the basic premise.

The research question was:

> What is the impact of this anxiety, aroused in parents in as early a stage as pregnancy, on their latent and overt emotional attitudes towards their sons, and relative to their parenting patterns?

In other words, what happens to this anxiety during the course of the son's life: Does it continue to exist in different ways? Does it penetrate the parenting patterns? And if so, what is its conscious manifestation, and how does it unconsciously manifest? What happens in Israeli parenting to sons? And primarily, are there aspects in Israeli parenting of which we are currently unaware?

How were the parents chosen?

In *quantitative* research, a random sample of a particular population is examined in a structured way to establish numerical data from which statistically reliable results can be derived that reflect the population as a whole.

However, this procedure is not suitable in *qualitative* research, the fundamental reasons being that the research is interested in delving into human emotions and thoughts rather than limiting itself only to answers that can be framed in numerical terms. The aim in qualitative research is to develop understandings and theoretical concepts from the narratives, repeatedly examining the conditions under which the theory exists (Miles & Huberman, 1994). When people are allowed to talk freely, without the limitations of structured guiding questions, a far greater scope of information is received, even when the sample is small. In this study, for example, the interviews themselves fill some 500 pages and, together with the analysis stages, total some 1,000 pages.

I initially contacted potential interviewees through a technique known as "snowballing". I asked everyone I thought might know parents in the appropriate age range who fulfil the research population criteria to put me in touch with them.

The criteria for choosing the parents

Between 2001 and 2003, I interviewed twelve couples in various meaningful junctures in their sons' lives: three couples were expecting the birth of a son; three couples had sons about to enter first grade; three couples had sons aged almost thirteen, which is the important bar mitzvah stage; and three couples had sons who would soon be recruited. These junctures in the lives of parents and sons were chosen since aspects of the sons' separation and development would naturally give rise to parental anxiety over their sons' lives—should such anxiety indeed accompany the course of child rearing.

Multiple variables influence the feelings surfacing around the issue of a son's recruitment. Since this is a new research subject, it was important to establish a picture that reflects, as far as possible, the impact of the knowledge of future recruitment on the parenting process, without the influence of other factors. I therefore sought to identify these factors and selected only parents who are *not* characterized by them:

» In a family that had already experienced the loss of an immediate family member (whether in military service or other circumstances), anxiety over the son's recruitment would likely be greater (and therefore the processes they would undergo relative to recruitment would be different) compared to that of *families who have not needed to cope with bereavement.*

» Parents of a son with a health problem that may prevent the son from being accepted for combat service would likely display a lower level of anxiety over the son's recruitment than that displayed by parents *of a son qualified for commando service.*

» The emotional reactions over the dangers of military service in parents who had not served in the army would inherently be driven by hearsay, unlike parents who had served and whose reactions therefore came from personal experience. Hence, those chosen were *parents who had served in the army.*

» Among Israeli-born parents, or parents who had immigrated to Israel as children, grew up with existential danger, and were raised on the value of risking their lives for the sake of the country, different feelings would likely surface while raising their son compared to those in parents from another culture with no existential threat or life-risking values who had immigrated at an older age. Hence, the study only included *parents who were Israeli-born or had immigrated to Israel before the age of ten.*

» It is likely that adoptive or foster parents would have a different emotional relationship with their son compared to that where *both parents are the son's biological parents.*

Additionally, since low socioeconomic-status parents might perceive the army as an opportunity for their son to move to a higher socioeconomic level, which would conflict with their anxiety over their son's life, the study included *only families of the socioeconomic middle class.* Finally, *all parents were Jewish and were between the ages of thirty and fifty-five.*

Among the interviewees, some had gone from high school into professional training, others held degrees or doctorates. Some were self-employed, others salaried. Professions included teaching, therapy, industry, and commerce. Their affinity to Judaism ranged from secular, to traditional, to religious. Some were city residents, some agricultural community members [*moshav*], and some cooperative agricultural community members [*kibbutz*]. Political views ranged from right-wing, to left-wing, to not clearly identified. Some lived within the "green line" area of Israel, some beyond it. Quite coincidentally, six of the couples had three boys each, and the other six couples also had girls. Equally coincidentally, in all families the number of sons was greater than the number of daughters. All couples I approached responded to my interview request warmly.

Conducting the interview

Most of the interviews were conducted in the parents' homes in the evening, when children were asleep or were out of the house; one couple was interviewed in the afternoon, as that was the most suitable time for them. All interviews were marked by quiet, private conversation. Interviewing both parents together also revealed information about their relationship.

I sought an interview method that would allow receiving personal, freely given reactions, including thoughts, intuitions, sensations, feelings, and insights, so that the data analysis and conclusions could be based on as full a picture as possible of the interviewees' current and past emotional expressions and behaviours at the conscious and unconscious levels. As is customary in qualitative psychological research, or in research of verbal history in the fields of psychology, history, and sociology (Gilligan, 1982; Lieblich, 1989; Lomsky-Feder, 1992), I chose *depth interviews and an open interview method* that allows listening with interest to what the parents have to say without directing or limiting them through specific questions. Focal open questions came up repeatedly in all interviews and allowed a free, unfacilitated conversation. This method enables accessing the interviewees' experiential and personal stances and allows room for the complexity existing in parents' feelings and relationships with their sons: the fluctuations, internal contradictions, ambivalences, and silences (Gilligan, 1982).

I opened the interviews by saying that I was interested in hearing "your thoughts and emotions about raising *children*". My question purposely did not mention sons specifically. I felt that if the son's future recruitment surfaces spontaneously in the interviews, it would indicate that the issue is indeed central to the parents' internal world. For me, the interview was a flexible tool that refined itself as the interview, and the developing dynamic, progressed (Mishler, 1986).

Up until this study, no attempt had been made in the world of research to explore social and familial phenomena. This meant that no previous knowledge was available on which I could base my work. For this reason, I tried to implement knowledge taken from the world of psychoanalysis, which focuses on unconscious processes. Of course, not all the psychoanalytic therapeutic principles were suited to this study, requiring me to audit and analyse the interviews by implementing the most *relevant psychoanalytic principles and understandings*.

The purpose of the interviews was defined in advance in a way that allowed the interviewees to feel throughout that I was interested in their psychic state and their emotions. During the course of the interviews, privacy and calm were maintained (Etchegoyen, 1991, pp. 86–126, 321–329). Unlike an analytic therapy session, no time limit was set for the interviews, allowing interviewees to express themselves freely.

Following the principles of psychotherapeutic and psychoanalytic frameworks, no personal details from my own life were provided during the interviews, to avoid distorting the couples' views. Unlike a therapy session, however, once interviewees had indicated they had said all they wished to say, I felt that certain details from my personal life would allow the interviewees to cope better with the emotional burdens that flooded them during the interview. The incidents I chose were based on considerations of how they might be meaningful for the interviewees. What mostly resurfaced were instances where I felt I could offer the parents some additional perspectives from my professional, research, and personal experience to legitimize their emotions expressed in the interviews and experienced by the parents as irregular or aberrant. In one case, for example, I told Dina, whose son was soon to be recruited, and who for the first time expanded on her anxieties, leaving her flooded by them, that I had also been anxious before my sons' recruitment, but once that is past and sons are in various training courses, there are many far lighter periods. With Leah, I shared the fact that most mothers participating in the study expressed similar feelings to hers, a statement she experienced as relief, saying "Oh, it's so good to know that I'm not the only crazy one." The degree of relief she felt manifested when she turned to her husband Lapid, repeating that statement: "See, Lapid? I'm not crazy . . ."

The reality in Israel during the period in which the interviews were conducted varied. The first four interviews were held during a period filled with a euphoric atmosphere, a sense that Israel was heading towards peace. The withdrawal from Lebanon was perceived as one link in a chain of diplomatic processes that commenced with the Oslo Accords in 1993 and the signing of a peace treaty with Jordan in 1994.

The remaining eight interviews, which began in November 2000, were conducted in an entirely different atmosphere: with the start of the Second Intifada, terror attacks hit the civilian population in Israel, and every week regular citizens, including children, were injured or killed. The previous euphoria was replaced by a feeling of lack of security. In April 2002, terrorists conducted a massacre on the eve of Passover in a packed-to-capacity hotel dining room, following which the Defensive Shield Operation took place, reconquering cities in which the terrorists were based, which had been transferred to the Palestinian Authority under the Oslo Agreement.

Irrespective of the level of tension around security in Israel, in all interviews the issue of the son's future recruitment occupied a significant part of the conversation and aroused intense emotions and internal conflicts, both interpersonal and between the couple, and shaped behaviours and plans into parental behavioural patterns that in part were concealed.

Being interested in the interviewees' unconscious worlds, and seeking to reconstruct the verbal and non-verbal messages as precisely as possible, the interviews were videoed and written up immediately after they were held, with descriptions of the body language accompanying the words.

Data analysis

In order to evaluate the unconscious processes, I used Gilligan's (1992) "voice-centred relational method". Wishing to evaluate the unconscious processes, I used this method to first audit a psychological study as detailed in "A Listener's Guide" (Brown & Gilligan, 1992).

The method focuses on listening to the interviewee's unique voice while paying attention to the voice's polyphonic spread, listening to the voice aroused in the interviewee during the interview, while documenting it, and while listening to the encounter between voices, and the dimension of the relationship being built between interviewer and interviewee. The *first stage* involves analysing the content while listening to the facts alone, without any interpretation, in terms of what is happening, and what is the sequence of events.

As the *second stage*, I employed the unique method of listening known as the "I-Poem", developed by Carol Gilligan (2002). It involves listing all instances where the word "I" appears, along with the verb immediately following it. These word pairs form a kind of poem; from their content, it is possible to feel which sentence closes each poem. In this way, many "I-Poems" were formed by each of the interviewed parents. This format makes it possible to listen to the basic verbs parents use when they speak about themselves, the packing of their speech, and the particular music each of them produces. "I-Poems" also provide an initial image of the interviewee's unique voice as well as how she or he relates to the self. In the findings, I occasionally use an "I-Poem" as a means of clarification.

The following example is from Yasmin's interview. From her remarks we might be impressed by how confident, talkative, and energetic she is, yet she also expresses doubts. But listening to the full text of her "I-Poem" reveals that the extent of her insecurity over her mothering is far greater than initial impressions would suggest. Since the scope of her difficulty is hidden from her surroundings, we might assume that Yasmin feels fairly alone with her difficulty. This is how her "I-Poem" looked, the first time I removed it from the full interview text:

I'm not a mother
I'm not pressured
When I hear
I'm not talking about the flu
I was also a sister
I'm totally not a pressured mother
I'm a crazy mother
I can go
I do damage
I think
I panic

Observing this when I removed it for the first time from the full text, I wondered why I had not stripped the entire text completely, the way Gilligan suggests doing. Suddenly I realized that the power of emotions being transmitted to me from within the exposed poem was so great that I needed to leave another word or two, to cover up its glaring nakedness. The more emotional manifestation provides some kind of relief; however, when I ignore most of these words following "I" it becomes possible to more powerfully sense the degree of difficulty Yasmin is concealing:

I'm not
I'm not
I hear
I'm not

I was
I'm totally not
I'm a mother
I can
I do
I think
I panic

Most of Yasmin's feelings around her mothering are that she "is not" and even "totally not". Even though she knows she "is a mother", that "she can" and that "she does", she feels this ambivalence and wonders about it—"I think". But in the end she is left in upheaval: "I panic."

In considering how to listen to the *couple voice* and evaluate the nature of a couple's parenting processes as a unit, and the couple's complex relationship dynamic, I developed a parallel "we-poem" technique, by extracting "we" sentences, which exposed the skeletal structure of the couple relationship.

For the *third stage*, data was analysed with "field anchored theory". I removed recurring topics from the texts and collected these motifs under one category while listening to key sentences, images, silences, internal contradictions, and reactions of the couple to each other's sentences, and paying attention to repetitive patterns in the couple relationship. Attention was also paid to disruptions to the flow of speech, such as slips of the tongue, momentary forgetfulness, distractions, etc. Relating to all these, according to Freud (1901), is to see them as expressing psychic actions and manifestations having content and meaning.

As I show below, the same motifs appeared in all the interviews. In the context of relevant psychoanalytic theories, several innovative theoretical understandings surfaced. In this way, a complex emotional picture began to emerge: the emotional and behavioural motifs typifying the interviewees, and the content and patterns typifying the relationships between parents and sons and between the parents themselves.

Data analysis based on the psychoanalytic approach

The interviewer's voice was detailed in the *fourth stage*, allowing a separation between the voices of the interviewees, and voices surfacing in me as the interviewer from within my own personal emotional material.

This stage was carried out after the interviews were reconstructed at the various levels when the unconscious emotional processes that a specific interview wrought in me were fully empowered, raw, without any processing that could evaluate their nature.

Wanting to raise at least some of the content to a conscious level, I started out, after completing these earlier stages, as though "turning a new leaf". I opened a new file in the computer and began writing whatever associatively surfaced. I tried to write down my thoughts, feelings, and associations without any interpretation or auditing. Sometimes I continued writing with my eyes closed, as though the content flowed by itself; sometimes I would find myself starting at the screen, and only after several minutes would I shake myself and realize I had not recorded what had happened inside me. Often, this path took me to my sons: my oldest who was discharged and, during the period in which I analysed the interviews, was traveling through Australia on a motorbike; my middle son, who was just beginning his military service in the Armoured Corps; and my youngest son, who was completing his senior-high-school studies and was approaching recruitment. Often I found my face wet with tears when acknowledging the pain that swept through me, getting lost in staring into empty space, wandering through the house as a means of escape when faced with emotions that, while functioning as the interviewer and performing rational analyses, I had held inside without any legitimate outlet.

I tried to cope, through self-analysis, assisted by psychoanalysis, as a place that allows emotional processing and greater consciousness. Later I sifted through specific content surfacing in myself, related to specific interviews, noting that when one interview raised certain content that others did not, it was a key to additional understandings. In this way, content of which I had been previously unconscious allowed me a better understanding of the complex emotional situations experienced by interviewees.

In the *fifth stage*, the encounter between the interviewees' voices and my own as the interviewer created the research understanding. The encounter between the stages allowed reaching understandings concerning the specific significances surfacing from the interview. During this stage, and most certainly when the process was completed for all interviews, the links among the relevant theories began to take shape; from within these links, new theoretical understandings consolidated.

REFERENCES

Almog, A. (1997). *The Sabra: The Creation of the New Jew*, trans. H. Watzman. Berkeley, CA: University of California Press, 2000.

Alshatien, H. (2014). *Children of War 1944–1948: Children Talk about the Holocaust.* Tel Aviv: Yediot Books. [In Hebrew]

Andrews, B., Brewin, C. R., Philpott, R., & Stewart, L. (2007). Delayed-onset post-traumatic stress disorder: A systematic review of the evidence. *American Journal of Psychiatry, 164*: 1319–1326.

Ashkenazi, A. (2010). Who are we talking about when we talk about PTSD: The simulacrum, trauma and responsibility. *Journal of Cinema and Television History (Jerusalem), 4*: 63-69. [In Hebrew]

Auerhahn, N. C., & Laub, D. (1998). The primal scene of atrocity. *Psychoanalytic Psychology, 15*: 360–377.

Bar-On, M. (1999). Securitism and critics: 1949–1967. In: M. Bar-On (Ed.), *Challenge the Sovereignty: Creation and Contemplation in the Country's First Decade.* Jerusalem: Yad Ben-Zvi.

Baudrillard, J. (1981). *Simulacra and Simulation.* Ann Arbor, MI: University of Michigan Press, 1994.

Ben-Ari, E. (1998). *Mastering Soldiers.* New York: Berghan Books.

Ben-Ari, E. (2001). Tests of soldierhood, trials of manhood: Military service and male ideals in Israel. In: D. Maman, E. Ben-Ari, & Z. Rosenhek (Eds.), *War, Politics and Society in Israel: Theoretical and Comparative Perspectives* (pp. 239–268). New Brunswick, NJ: Transaction Publishers.

Ben-Ari, E., & Levy-Schreiber, E. (2000). Body-building, character-building and nation-building: Gender and military service in Israel. *Studies in Contemporary Judaism, 16*: 171–190.

Ben-Ariea, Y., & Reiner, E. (2003). *In Judah: Studies in the History Land. Israel and Settlement.* Jerusalem: Yad Ben-Tzvi. [In Hebrew]

Benjamin, J. (1995). *Like Subjects, Love Objects: Essays on Recognition and Sexual* Difference (pp. 27–48). New Haven, CT: Yale University Press.

Bion, W. R. (1959). Attacks on linking. *International Journal of Psychoanalysis, 40*: 308–315. Reprinted in: *Second Thoughts.* London: Heinemann.

Bion, W. R. (1967). *Second Thoughts.* London: Heinemann.

Bion, W. R. (1997). *War Memoirs 1917–1919*, ed. F. Bion. London: Karnac.
Block, J. H. (1973). Conception of sex role: Some cross-cultural and longitudinal perspectives. *American Psychologist, 23*: 339–340.
Blos, P. (1962). *On Adolescence*. New York: Free Press.
Blos, P. (1967). The second individuation process of adolescence. *Psychoanalytic Study of the Child, 22*: 162–186.
Boni, N. (2012). The secular pilgrim. *Internal Security*, 2 November.
Bowlby, J. (1988). Caring for children. In: *A Secure Base: Clinical Applications of Attachment* (pp. 1–22). London: Routledge.
Brenner, I. (2014). *Dark Matters: Exploring the Realm of Psychic Devastation*. London: Karnac.
Brown, L. M., & Gilligan, C. (1992). A listener's guide In: *Meeting at the Crossroads: Women's Psychology and Girls' Development*. Cambridge, MA: Harvard University Press.
Chetrit-Vatine, V. (2014). *The Analyst's Ethical Awakening: Levinas's Philosophy as a Contemporary Psychoanalysis*. Paper presented at the International Psychoanalytic University, Berlin, 18 September.
Chodorow, N. J. (1978). Gender differences in the preoedipal period. *The Reproduction of Mothering: Psychoanalysis and the Sociology of Gender* (pp. 92–139). Berkeley, CA: University of California Press.
Deleuze, G., & Guattari, F. (1975). *Kafka: Toward a Minor Literature*. Theory and History of Literature, Vol. 30. Minneapolis, MN: University of Minnesota Press, 1986.
Dicks, H. (1967). *Marital Tension*. London: Routledge & Kegan Paul.
Elitzur, A. (2003). *A Dream of Freud's in Light of Rotenberg's Attitude to Psychoanalysis*. Available [in Hebrew] at: http://a-c-elitzur.co.il/site/siteArticle.asp?ar=122
Erikson, E. H. (1950). *Childhood and Society*. New York: Norton, 1962.
Erlich, H. S. (1990). Boundaries, limitations, and the wish for fusion in the treatment of adolescents. *Psychoanalytic Study of the Child, 45*: 195–213.
Erlich, H. S. (1998). On loneliness, narcissism, and intimacy. *American Journal of Psychoanalysis, 58* (2): 135–162.
Esman, A. E. (1985). Discussion: Paternal hostility and parental ambivalence. *International Journal of Psychoanalytic Psychotherapy, 11*: 145–148.
Etchegoyen, E. (1991). *The Fundamentals of Psychoanalytic Technique*. London: Karnac.
Faimberg, H. (2005). *The Telescoping of Generations: Listening to the Narcissistic Links between Generations*. London: Routledge & the Institute of Psychoanalysis.
Fairbairn, W. R. D. (1944). Endopsychic structure considered in terms of object relationships. *International Journal of Psychoanalysis, 25*: 70–92.

Reprinted in: *Psychoanalytic Studies of the Personality* (pp. 82–136). London: Tavistock, 1952.

Fairbairn, W. R. D. (1952). *Psychoanalytic Studies of the Personality.* London: Tavistock.

Fairbairn, W. R. D. (1963). Synopsis of an object-relations theory of the personality. *International Journal of Psychoanalysis, 44*: 224–225.

Freud, A. (1936). The ego and the id at puberty. In: *The Ego and the Mechanisms of Defense* (pp. 137–151). New York: International Universities Press, 1958.

Freud, A., & Burlingham, D. (1942). *War and Children.* New York: International Universities Press.

Freud, S. (1895) (with Breuer, J.). *Studies on Hysteria. Standard Edition, 2*: 1–319.

Freud, S. (1900). *The Interpretation of Dreams. Standard Edition, 4/5.*

Freud, S. (1901). *The Psychology of Everyday Life. Standard Edition, 6.*

Freud, S. (1905). *Three Essays on the Theory of Sexuality. Standard Edition, 7*: 125–245.

Freud, S. (1912–13). *Totem and Taboo. Standard Edition, 13*: 1–161.

Freud, S. (1914). Remembering, repeating and working-through (Further recommendations on the technique of psycho-analysis II). *Standard Edition, 12*: 145–156.

Freud, S. (1915a). Instincts and their vicissitudes. *Standard Edition, 14*: 111–140.

Freud, S. (1915b). A case of paranoia running counter to the psycho-analytic theory of the disease. *Standard Edition, 14*: 261–272.

Freud, S. (1915c). Thoughts for the times on war and death. *Standard Edition, 14*: 273–300.

Freud, S. (1915d). Repression. *Standard Edition, 14*: 141–158.

Freud, S. (1919). Introduction to *Psycho-Analysis and the War Neuroses. Standard Edition, 19*: 205–216.

Freud, S. (1920). *Beyond the Pleasure Principle. Standard Edition, 18*: 1–64.

Freud, S. (1921). *Group Psychology and the Analysis of the Ego. Standard Edition, 18*: 65–144.

Freud, S. (1923). *The Ego and the Id. Standard Edition, 19*: 1–66.

Freud, S. (1925). Negation. *Standard Edition, 19*: 233–240.

Freud, S. (1933). Why war? *Standard Edition, 22*: 195–216.

Freud, S. (1939). *Moses and Monotheism. Standard Edition, 23*: 1–138.

Friedlander, S. (1983). *Nazi Germany and the Jews: 1933-1939.* Tel Aviv: Am-Oved. [In Hebrew]

Gampel, Y. (2005). *The Parents Who Live through Me.* Jerusalem: Keter. [In Hebrew]

Gan, A. (2009). *The Tanks of Tammuz* and *The Seventh Day*: The emergence of opposite poles of Israeli identity after the Six Day War. *Journal of Israeli History, 28* (2): 155–173.

Gilligan, C. (1982). *In a Different Voice*. Cambridge, MA: Harvard University Press.

Gilligan, C. (2002). *The Birth of Pleasure*. New York: Alfred A. Knopf.

Gould, R. (1975). Adult life stages: A growth towards self tolerance. *Psychology Today, 8* (9): 74–78.

Green, A. (1975). The analyst, symbolization and absence in the analytic setting (On changes in analytic practice and analytic experience). *International Journal of Psychoanalysis, 56*: 1–22.

Guvrin, N. (1935). Remote flesh: The responses to the Holocaust in Hebrew literature of those who were there. *North: Literary File, Haifa, 4*: 209–230. [In Hebrew]

Hadari, I. (2002). *Messiah Rides a Tank: Public Thought Between the Sinai Campaign and the Yom Kippur War 1955–1975*. Tel Aviv: Hakibbutz Hamuhad.

Harel, A. (2013). *Every Hebrew Mother Will: Portrait of the New Army*. Galilee: Zamora-Dvir.

Hever, H., & Ron, M. (Eds.) (1983). *Fighting and Killing without End: Political Poetry in the Lebanon War*. Tel Aviv: Hakibbutz Hamuhad.

Hughes, R. (1961). *The Fox in the Attic*. London: Chatto & Windus.

Hunter, F. T., & Youniss, J. (1982). Changes in functions of three relations in adolescence. *Developmental Psychology, 18*: 806–811.

Ibsen, H. (1865). Letter to Björnstjerne Björnson. In: *Letters of Henrik Ibsen*, trans. J. N. Laurvik & M. Morison. New York: Fox, Duffield and Co, 1905.

Isachar, H. (2003). *Feminist Voices of the Left*. Fetish: An Israeli Series for Cultural Studies. Tel Aviv: Resling. [In Hebrew]

Jacobus, M. (2005). Magical arts: The poetics of play. *Psychoanalytic History, 7*: 21–50.

Jones, E. (1957). *Sigmund Freud. Life and Work, Vol. 3: The Last Phase 1919–1939*. London: Hogarth Press.

Klein, M. (1937a). A contribution to the psychogenesis of manic-depressive states. In: *Love, Guilt & Reparation and Other Works 1921*–1945 (pp. 262–289). London: Hogarth Press, 1975.

Klein, M. (1937b). Love, guilt and reparation. In: *Love, Guilt and Reparation and Other Works* (pp. 306–343). London: Hogarth Press, 1975.

Klein, M. (1946). Notes on some schizoid mechanisms. In: M. Klein, P. Heimann, S. Isaacs & J. Riviere, *Developments in Psychoanalysis* (pp. 292–320). London: Hogarth Press, 1975.

Kogan, E. (1995). Love and the heritage of the past. *International Journal of Psycho-Analysis, 76*: 805–824.

Kohlberg, L., & Gilligan, C. (1972). The adolescent as a philosopher: The discovery of the self in a post-conventional world. In: J. Kagan & R. Coles (Eds.), *12 to 16: Early Adolescence*. New York: Norton.

Kolonimus, N. L., & Bar-Tal, D. (2011). Perception of the conflict ethos and the military service among elite units' soldiers. *The Public Space, Internet Journal*. [Department of Political Science, Tel Aviv University.]

Lacan, J. (1956). On a question prior to any possible treatment of psychosis. In: *Écrits: The First Complete Edition in English* (pp. 445–448). New York: Norton, 2002.

Laplanche, J., & Pontalis, J.-B. (1973). *The Language of Psycho-Analysis*. London: Karnac, 1988.

Laub, D. (1998). The empty circle: Children of survivors and the limits of reconstruction. *Journal of the American Psychoanalytic Association, 46*: 507–529.

Laub, D., & Lee, S. (2003). Thanatos and massive psychic trauma: The impact of the death instinct on knowing, remembering and forgetting. *Journal of the American Psychoanalytic Association, 51*: 433–463.

Lau-Lavie, N. (1993). *The Nation as a Lion: An Autobiography*. Jerusalem: Keter. [In Hebrew]

Layland, R. (1985). In search of a loving father. In: A. Samuels (Ed.), *The Father: Contemporary Jungian Perspectives* (pp. 154–169). London: Free Association Books.

Levi, I. (2003). *The Other Army of Israel: Materialist Militarism in Israel*. Tel Aviv: Miscal Publishing House, Yediot Acharonot and Hemed Library. [In Hebrew]

Levi, I. (2004). Cure in Bubo Way: Reading in Freud's mythological parallel to a visual obsession. *Sihot, 18* (2): 135–146. [In Hebrew]

Levi, I., Witztum, A., Granek, M., & Kotler, M. (1989). Combat reaction in Israel's wars from 1948 to 1973, Part I: Background and history, methodology and a review of the literature of the period. *Sihot, 4* (1): 60–70.

Levi, P. (1963). *If This Is a Man & The Truce*. London: Abacus.

Levinston, D. J. (1986). A conception of adult development. *American Psychologist, 4*: 3–13.

Lewow, E. (2004). Negation of time and reality: Thoughts on parenthood without boundaries. In: E. Perroni (Ed.), *Time Psychoanalysis and Other Disciplines* (pp. 39–51). Tel Aviv: Hakibbutz Hameuchad. [In Hebrew]

Lewow, E. (2011). *Parenting From Another Direction: An Experimental Publishing*. Jerusalem. [In Hebrew]

Lewow, E. (in press). *Where Are You? From Disorientation to Growth-Fostering Parenting*. Tel Aviv: Modan. [In Hebrew]

Liebes, T., & Blum-Kulka, S. (1994). Managing a moral dilemma: Israeli soldiers in the Intifada. *Armed Forces & Society, 21* (1): 45–68.

Lieblich, A. (1989). *Transition to Adulthood during Military Service: The Israeli Case* (pp. 181–195). Albany, NY: SUNY Press.

Lieblich, A. (2001). Mother–son relationships in the shadow of war. In: A. O'Reilly (Ed.), *Mothers and Sons: Feminism, Masculinity, and the Struggle to Raise Our Sons* (pp. 235–250). London: Routledge.

Lisak, M., & Kimmerling, B. (Eds.) (1984). *Military and Security: A Reader.* Jerusalem: The Hebrew University. [In Hebrew]

Loewald., H. W. (2000) The waning of the Oedipus complex. *Journal of Psychotherapy Practice and Research, 9* (4): 239–249.

Lomsky-Feder, E. (1992). Youth in the shadow of war—War in the light of youth: Life-stories of Israeli veterans. In: *Adolescence, Careers, and Cultures* (pp. 393–408). New York: Walter de Gruyter.

Lomsky-Feder, E., & Ben-Ari, E. (1999). Introduction: Cultural constructions of war and the military in Israel. In: E. Lomsky-Feder & E. Ben-Ari (Eds.), *The Military and Militarism in Israeli Society*. Albany, NY: SUNY Press.

Luski, H. D. (2001). The Rizum thinking. In: *Resling: A Multidisciplinary Stage for Culture, 8:* 12–24. [In Hebrew]

Lyotard, J. F. (1988). *Heidegger and the Jews.* Minnesota, MN: The Regents of the University of Minnesota, 1990.

Mailer, N. (1948). *The Naked and the Dead.* New York: Rinehart & Co.

Mann-Shalvi, H. (2005). *From Ultrasound to the Draft: The Impact of the Knowledge That Boys in Israel Are Drafted at Eighteen on the Conscious and Unconscious Emotional Attitudes and Relatedness of their Parents.* Doctoral thesis, the Hebrew University of Jerusalem. [In Hebrew]

Mann-Shalvi, H. (2007a). Germans and Israeli Jews: Hidden emotional dynamics In: H. Parens, A. Mahfouz, S. Twemlow, & D. Scharff (Eds.), *The Future of Prejudice: Psychoanalysis and the Prevention of Prejudice* (pp. 255–268). Lanham, MD: Aronson.

Mann-Shalvi, H. (2007b). *The Influence of Military Service on the Conscious and Unconscious Emotional Attitude, Identity and Functioning of the Israeli-born Soldier.* Proposed research plan presented to the IPA Postgraduate Centre for Psychoanalytic Studies, 13th Annual Research Training Programme, London, 2–10 August.

Mann-Shalvi, H. (2010). *Three Minds, One Space (TMOS): Combined Emotional of the Couple and Their Link.* Paper presented at the 4th Conference of the International Association of Couple and Family Psychoanalysis, Buenos Aires, Argentina.

Meadow, P. W., & Green, A. (2006). Freud and modern psychoanalysis: A discussion. *Modern Psychoanalysis, 31*: 7–24.

Mevorach, O. (1977). *The Long Trip after the Military Service: Characteristics of the Travellers, the Effect of the Trip, and Its Meaning*. Doctoral dissertation, the Hebrew University of Jerusalem. [In Hebrew]

Miles, M. B., & Huberman, A. M. (1994). *Qualitative Data Analysis* (2nd edition). Beverly Hills, CA: Sage.

Milo, H. (2012). *Songs Speak: Identity, Gender, and Ideology in Songs of Israeli Soldiers.* Doctoral thesis, University of Haifa. [In Hebrew]

Mishler, E. G. (1986). The analysis of interview narratives. In: T. R. Sarbin (Ed.), *Narrative Psychology* (pp. 233–255). New York: Praeger.

Morman, M. T., & Floyd, K. (2002). A changing culture of fatherhood: Effects on affectionate communication, closeness, and satisfaction in men's relationships with their fathers and their sons. *Western Journal of Communication, 66* (4): 395–411.

Nadelson, T. (2005). *Trained to Kill: Soldiers at War*. Baltimore, MD: Johns Hopkins University Press.

Nietzsche, F. (1872). *The Birth of Tragedy: Out of the Spirit of Music*, trans. S. Whiteside, ed. M. Tanner. London: Penguin, 1994.

Nora, P. (1993). Between memory and history: On a problem of the place. *Zmanim, 7* (4): 45. [In Hebrew]

Noy, C. (2007). *A Narrative Community: Voices of Israeli Backpackers.* Detroit, IL: Wayne State University Press.

Ofrat, G. (2004). *Within a Local Context*. Tel Aviv: Hakibbutz Hameuchad. [In Hebrew]

Ogden, T. H. (1989). *The Primitive Edge of Experience.* Northvale, NJ: Aronson.

Ogden, T. H. (1994). *Subjects of Analysis.* London: Karnac.

Ogden, T. H. (2014). Fear of breakdown and the unlived life. *International Journal of Psychoanalysis, 95*: 205–223.

Palgi-Hecker, A. (2005). *Mothers in Psychoanalysis: A Feminist View.* Tel Aviv: Am Oved.

Parker, R. (1996). *Torn in Two.* London: Virago.

Pelach-Galil, R. (2004). *Fathers and Adolescent Boys.* Doctoral thesis, Hebrew University of Jerusalem. [In Hebrew]

Peterson, G. W., & Steinmetz, S. K. (2000). The diversity of fatherhood: Change, constancy, and contradiction. *Marriage and Family Review, 29* (4): 315–322.

Reeves, C. (2004). On being "intrinsical": A Winnicott enigma. *American Imago, 61*: 427–455.

Rotenberg, M. (2003). In the name of the father, the son and the goblin. In: *Midrash Mind: Studies in Psychology and Judaism in Honour of Mordechai Rotenberg*. Tel Aviv: Yediot Aharonot.

Rubin-Sagi, A. (1998). Proud Hebraic soldier wants to go home. *Ototot, 98* (218): 32–33, 50–51. [In Hebrew].

Sasson-Levy, O. (2006) *Identities in Uniform: Masculinities and Femininities in the Israeli Military*. The Eshkolot Library, The Levey Eshkol Institute. Jerusalem: The Hebrew University Magnes Press. [In Hebrew]

Sayers, J. (1991). *Mothering Psychoanalysis*. Harmondsworth: Penguin, 2000.

Scharff, J. S., & Scharff, D. E. (2011) The link. In: *The Interpersonal Unconscious* (pp. 23–39). Lanham, MD: Aronson.

Scharff, J. S., & Scharff, D. E. (Eds.) (2014). *Psychoanalytic Couple Therapy: Foundations of Theory and Practice*. London: Karnac.

Schweid, E. (1990). *Wrestling Until Daybreak*. Tel Aviv: Hakibutz Hameuhad. [In Hebrew]

Segev, T. (1991). *The Seventh Million: The Israelis and the Holocaust*. Jerusalem: Maxwell-Maximilian Keter.

Segev, T. (2007). *1967: Israel, the War, and the Year That Transformed the Middle East*. New York: Henry Holt.

Shabtai, A. (2000). *Greek Mythology, Myths*. Tel Aviv: Mapa. [In Hebrew]

Shafir, G., & Peled, Y. (1998). Citizenship and stratification in an ethnic democracy. In: *Ethnic and Racial Studies, 21* (3): 408–428.

Shalvi, E. (2016). *Changes in Soldiers' Images During Sixty Years from 1948 in the Military Weekly Journal Bamakhaneh*. Doctoral thesis, Ben-Gurion University (in preparation).

Shapira, A. (1967). *The Seventh Day: Soldiers Talk about the Six-Day War*. London: Simon & Schuster, 1971.

Shapira, A. (1997). *New Jews, Old Jews*. Ofakim Library. Tel Aviv: Am Oved. [In Hebrew]

Shatan, C. F. (1977). Bogus manhood, bogus honor. *Psychoanalytic Review, 64* (4): 586–610.

Sheely, G. (1976). *Passages: Predictable Crises of Adult Life*. New York: Dutton.

Shinoda-Bolen, J. (2002). *Gods in Everyman*. Ben Shemne: Modan. [In Hebrew]

Shoham, S. G. (1998). Tantalus processes. In: *Personality Theory* (pp. 241–254). Tel-Aviv: Tcherikover.

Shoham, S. G. (2005). The Binding of Isaac. In: *The Myth of Tantalus: A Scaf-*

folding for an Ontological Personality Theory. Brighton: Sussex University Press.

Shulman, S., & Seiffge-Krenke, I. (1997). *Fathers and Adolescents: Developmental and Clinical Perspectives*. New York: Routledge.

Silverman, L. H. (1982). *The Search for Oneness*. New York: International Universities Press.

Slater, M. D., Henry, K. L., Swaim, A. R., & Anderson, L. L. (2003). Violent media content and aggressiveness in adolescents. *Communication Research, 30* (6): 713–736.

Slavin, M., & Kriegman, D. (1992). *The Adaptive Design of the Human Psyche: Psychoanalysis, Evolutionary Biology, and the Therapeutic Process*. New York: Guilford Press.

Solomon, Z. (1993). *Combat Stress Reaction: The Enduring Toll of War*. New York: Plenum Press.

Solomon, Z., Lev-Shalem, L., & Dekel, R. (2007). The link between exposure to a traumatic event, developing PTSD and perceptions of soldiers who fought in the Yom Kippur War. *Trends: Journal of Interdisciplinary Social Sciences, 4*: 690–706.

Solomon, Z., & Mikulincer, M. (2006). Trajectories of PTSD: A 20-year longitudinal study. *American Journal of Psychiatry, 163* (4): 659–666.

Steir-Livny, L. (2011). The threefold exile: The female Holocaust survivor in Israeli cinema. In: M. Shilo & G. Katz (Eds.), *Gender in Israel: New Studies on Gender in the Yishuv and the State* (pp. 497–522). Iyunim bitkumat Israel Thematic Series, 6. Seder Boker: Ben-Gurion Research Institute. [In Hebrew]

Sullivan, H. S. (1953). *The Interpersonal Theory of Psychiatry*. New York: Norton.

Tal, K. J. (1991). *Bearing Witness: The Literature of Trauma*. New Haven, CT: Yale University Press.

Target, M., & Fonagy, P. (2002). Fathers in modern psychoanalysis and in society: The role of the father and child. In: J. Trowell & A. Etchegoyen (Eds.), *The Importance of Fathers: A Psychoanalytic Re-Evaluation* (pp. 41–66). Hove: Brunner Routledge.

Teveth, S. (1968). *The Tanks of Tammuz*. London: Weidenfeld & Nicolson.

Volkan, V. D. (2012). The intertwining of the internal and external wars. In: M. Gerard Fromm (Ed.), *Lost in Transmission: Studies of Trauma across Generations*. London: Karnac.

Volkan, V. D., & Greer, W. F. Jr. (2002). *The Third Reich in the Unconscious: Transgenerational Transmission and Its Consequences*. New York: Brunner-Routledge.

Winnicott, C. (1990). D.W.W: A reflection. In: P. Giovacchini (Ed.), *Tactics and Techniques in Psychoanalytic Therapy, Vol. 3: The Implications of Winnicott's Contributions* (pp. 3–20). London: Aronson.

Winnicott, D. W. (1940). Discussion of war aims. In: *Home Is Where We Start From: Essays by a Psychoanalyst* (pp. 210–220). New York: Norton, 1986.

Winnicott, D. W. (1956). Primary maternal preoccupations. In: *Collected Papers: Through Paediatrics to Psycho-*Analysis (pp. 300–305). London: Tavistock, 1958.

Winnicott, D. W. (1960). Ego distortion in terms of true and false self. In: *The Maturational Processes and the Facilitating Environment* (pp. 140–152). London: Hogarth Press, 1965.

Winnicott, D. W. (1962). Ego integration in child development. In: *The Maturational Processes and the Facilitating Environment* (pp. 56–63). London: Hogarth Press, 1965.

Winnicott, D. W. (1963). Fear of breakdown. In: *Psycho-Analytic Explorations* (pp. 87–95), ed. C. Winnicott, R. Shepherd, & M. Davis. London: Karnac, 1989.

Winnicott, D. W. (1968). The use of the object and relating through identifications. In: *Playing and Reality* (pp. 86–94). London: Routledge, 1971.

Winnicott, D. W. (1969). The mother–infant experience of mutuality. In: *Psycho-Analytic Explorations* (pp. 251–260), ed. C. Winnicott, R. Shepherd, & M. Davis. London: Karnac, 1989.

Winnicott, D. W. (1971). *Playing and Reality,* London: Routledge.

Yehuda, R., McFarlane, A. C., & Shalev, A. Y. (1998). Predicting the development of posttraumatic stress disorder from the acute response to a traumatic event. *Biological Psychiatry, 44*: 1305–1313.

Yerushalmi, H. (1997). A psychoanalytic perspective on late adolescence in men in an Israeli combat unit. *Psychoanalytic Psychology, 14*: 113–127.

Yerushalmi, H. (2008). The endurance of the unstable. *Psychoanalytic Psychology, 25*: 309–325.

Yogman, M. W. (1982). Observations on the father–infant relationship. In: S. H. Cath, A. R. Gurwitt, & J. M. Ross (Eds.), *Father and Child: Developmental and Clinical Perspectives* (pp. 101–122). Boston, MA: Little Brown.

Young, I. M. (1990). *Throwing Like a Girl and Other Essays in Feminist Philosophy and Social Theory.* Bloomington, IN: Indiana University Press.

Zilberstein, T. (2013). *Soldiers Must Do So: The Israeli Soldier's Image in Israeli Theatre and Cinema.* Tel Aviv: Resling. [In Hebrew]

Zuckerman, M. (2001). *Israeli Factories: Myths and Ideology in Conflict.* Tel Aviv: Resling. [In Hebrew]

INDEX

For Product Safety Concerns and Information please contact our EU representative GPSR@taylorandfrancis.com Taylor & Francis Verlag GmbH, Kaufingerstraße 24, 80331 München, Germany

Batch number: 10725937

Printed by Printforce, the Netherlands